Personal Development Plans for Dentists

The new approach to continuing professional development

Amar Rughani
Associate Dean for Postgraduate Medical Education
University of Sheffield

with

Chris Franklin
Regional Postgraduate Dean
School of Clinical Dentistry
University of Sheffield

and

Stephen Dixon
Associate Dental Dean for CPD
South Yorkshire and East Midlands

Forewords by
Dame Margaret Seward and John Renshaw

Radcliffe Medical Press

Radcliffe Medical Press Ltd
18 Marcham Road
Abingdon
Oxon OX14 1AA
United Kingdom

www.radcliffe-oxford.com
The Radcliffe Medical Press electronic catalogue and online ordering facility.
Direct sales to anywhere in the world.

British Library Cataloguing in Publication Data

A catalogue record for this book is available from the British Library.

ISBN 1 85775 917 6

Typeset by Joshua Associates Ltd, Oxford
Printed and bound by TJ International Ltd, Padstow, Cornwall

Contents

Foreword

We are often reassuringly told that to learn from our mistakes is experience! While this may be so, it is only satisfying if the event is reflected upon, the lessons learnt and, more importantly, changes to practice take place so as to prevent repeat occurrences. What is often forgotten is the reverse side of the coin and that it is equally important to reflect on and learn from the successful events when everything went according to plan: truly a confidence-building exercise.

Plans have their rightful place in today's culture of life-long learning. It is fundamental not only to identify our current level of learning and professional competence, but also to identify areas for future development, so broadening our horizons and expertise. Personal development plans achieve this and, although flexibly constructed, will ensure that valuable learning and reflective time is used to best effect and for the ultimate benefit of our patients.

Recertification has been a great success story for the dental profession. The consultation document circulated by the General Dental Council in 1997 met with strong support for the principles in the Scheme, so it was not surprising that the uptake of the Voluntary GDC Scheme in 2000, in the absence of legislation, exceeded all expectations. Now, as we enter the era of mandatory recertification or CPD and the exploration of revalidation and appraisal for practitioners, the method of recognising and recording learning events is critical.

There will also be the need to understand the burgeoning terminology and array of acronyms accompanying CPD. Two deserve to be committed to memory – PUNs (Patients' Unmet Needs) and DENs (Dentist's Educational Needs). Any mismatch signals shortcomings in the dental practitioner's range of skills and techniques which in the past may have conveniently been blamed on the failings of our patients!

It will be relatively easy for most GDPs to sign up on sufficient approved courses of activity to satisfy the verifiable 75 hours of CPD in a five-year cycle. More challenging will be the task of how to ensure that the remaining 175 hours of non-verifiable activity is spent productively. Fortunately, help is at hand for the busy practitioner in the form of this excellent and immensely readable guide by Amar Rughani, and collaborating authors Chris Franklin and Stephen Dixon, who are all well-known enthusiasts and communicators in the field of professional development.

Nevertheless, this book is not intended as a comfortable armchair read! This guide is packed with down-to-earth sensible advice, interactive checkpoints to stimulate discussion and blank proformas which can be downloaded from the Internet for individual participation.

Personal Development Plans for Dentists is guaranteed to inspire as well as educate and deserves to be a 'must buy' for all dentists.

Dame Margaret Seward
Former President of the General Dental Council
Former Chief Dental Officer, England
January 2003

Foreword

Dear Dentist

The issue of professional revalidation and quality assurance has become something of an enigma. The jargon words and catch-phrases associated with this blossoming area of activity are bandied about with little concern for their real meaning, and practitioners at the bar regularly pontificate at length on this subject with little apparent grasp of the concepts that underlie the topic.

The need for a practical guide to the whole area of clinical governance and its many component parts, especially the Personal Development Plan (PDP), has been with us for a long time and at last an answer has been provided. This book is the answer to the caring dentist's demand for a thoughtful but essentially pragmatic approach to the use of quality control in a busy clinical setting – the nuts and bolts, the blueprint, of building your very own PDP.

When I was asked to write the foreword to this book I was immediately intrigued. I have seen one or two other attempts that have come close to the average dentist's requirements but this one appears to me to be just about spot on. It has everything to take you from basic comprehension of what is being asked of you right through to a full understanding of what participation in professional appraisal is all about, what it is meant to achieve and what you as an individual should gain from it.

In today's consumer society, the need for clinical quality assurance could be perceived by some as an externally imposed nightmare. The reality is that quality assurance has been practised for decades but it has not been formally structured nor has it been called by its various fashionable names. The right of the patient to be reassured that the professional providing care for them is up to date and capable of doing his or her job seems to me to be a 'given', any objection to their demands can only be seen as perverse. The truth is that conscientious professionals have always taken care to maintain their professional competence; the Personal Development Plan is the tool by which that activity can be structured and by which the level of activity can be demonstrated to an inquisitive third party, if that becomes necessary.

Amar Rughani and his collaborating authors claim that the Personal Development Plan is the cornerstone of clinical governance and, having read this book, I am certain they are right. This book will walk you through the whole process and show you exactly how to create your own PDP and how to deliver its contents for the benefit of you and your patients.

Best of luck!

John Renshaw
Chairman, BDA Executive Board
January 2003

Preface

The face of continuing professional development (CPD) for health professionals is changing rapidly, spurred on by societal pressures for accountability and the professions' need to periodically review fitness to practise. Once a private affair, CPD used to be little more than the responsibility of the individual to keep up to date. Nowadays, the emphasis is on the application of learning rather than just its acquisition and on the development of the dental team as much as the individual.

Over the past few years, personal development plans (PDPs) have been introduced for general medical practitioners and, with the encouragement of the educational community, they have become the main outcome of a formative appraisal process. The revalidation process, on which the licence to practise of doctors and dentists depends, is currently being formulated. For doctors, the practitioner's PDP and the associated evidence of learning will be a vital feature and it is likely that this will also be the case for dentists.

The acceptance of evidence-based education as the hallmark of professional competence is to be welcomed, especially as the alternative was prescriptive performance review. However, the implications of this are poorly understood by those who will have to engage with it.

At the heart of the new CPD will be the dentist's personal development plan, and in this book, the educational principles behind it are explained and illustrated. To develop a PDP and use the techniques that enrich it is to understand how and why dental CPD is moving forward. In doing so, dentists should experience the benefits that reflective practice can bring to patient care and self-esteem and thereby feel that they are willingly in step on the road ahead.

Amar Rughani
January 2003

This is a practical text and throughout the book, blank templates of the forms used are presented at the end of each chapter for your use – they can also be downloaded from the Internet at www.radcliffe-oxford.com/pdpdentists.

About the author

Amar Rughani is a GP in a large suburban practice in Sheffield and is Associate Dean for Postgraduate Medical Education for the South Yorkshire and South Humber Deanery. His expertise in the determinants of professional performance derives from his work as an examiner for the Royal College of General Practitioners (RCGP) and from personal experience of having completed Fellowship by Assessment (FBA) of the RCGP. His main role is in developing the principles of continuing professional development and supporting his colleagues in applying them to practice.

In recent years, he has worked collaboratively with his dental colleagues in the region to develop a reflective and formative approach to postgraduate dental education. Importantly, as a full-time general practitioner as well as an educationalist, his knowledge of what is achievable rather than just what is desirable has helped general dental practitioners (GDPs) to embrace the changes. As a result, GDPs have been able to demonstrate that, with a professional approach to education, improvements to practice can be generated more successfully from within than when they are imposed from without.

About the contributors

Dr Chris Franklin BDS, FDSRCS, PhD, FRCPath is Regional Postgraduate Dental Dean for South Yorkshire and East Midlands (formerly Trent NHSE), as well as a clinical academic and Honorary NHS Consultant in Histopathology (Oral and Maxillofacial Pathology). He has wide experience in undergraduate and postgraduate education and was a long-standing examiner for the Royal College of Surgeons, England for the primary and final Fellowship in Dental Surgery. Previous appointments include Hospital Dental Tutor and Regional Faculty Advisor for the Royal College of Surgeons, England. He is currently National CPD Advisor for his speciality at the Royal College of Pathologists. In 2000, he was instrumental in establishing the *CPD Dentistry Journal* and is currently involved in the development of a curriculum and clinical competencies for SHOs in dentistry.

Dr Stephen Dixon BDS, MFGDP(UK) is Associate Postgraduate Dental Dean for CPD for South Yorkshire and East Midlands (formerly Trent NHSE), as well as a general dental practitioner. He has been involved in vocational training for over 12 years. He was until recently a Postgraduate Dental Tutor for Grimsby and Scunthorpe. He lectures with Professor Robert Yemm on complete denture replacements.

Over the last two years, the contributors have been working with Postgraduate Dental Tutors, Vocational Training Advisors and colleagues such as Amar Rughani to encourage dental practitioners in the region to use PDPs as part of their clinical governance process and in working towards their requirements for recertification.

Acknowledgements

Although I am confident of my area of expertise, this book would neither have been credible or as readable if it were not for the contribution of the following dental colleagues with whom I have worked in the past few years in South Yorkshire and the East Midlands. Their talent, support and inspiration have shown me first-hand the value of collaboration between the professions. When it comes to education and the desire to improve, we are all brothers under the skin.

I would particularly like to thank: Dr Stephen Dixon, Dr Chris Franklin, Dr Simon Lidster and his colleagues in the Hillsborough group, Dr Laurence Jacobs, Dr John Skelton, Dr Lee Worthington, Dr Stephen Ellis, Dr Asha Ellis, Benjamin Dixon and Dr Stephen Fayle.

Amar Rughani
January 2003

In loving memory of my mother
Dr Gargi Rughani
29/11/26–6/4/02

1 About learning

Key points

- Many dentists were never taught or shown how to learn.
- We need to think less about acquiring information and more about applying what we learn.
- Revalidation will require us to demonstrate our learning.
- Being able to admit our shortcomings is the first step to self-improvement.
- Time spent educating ourselves is as valuable as time spent treating patients.
- Most experiences can begin a learning cycle.
- Even before we create time, we must protect the time we currently have for reflection.
- We can study the changes we have made to our practice to determine how best to learn.
- Participating, evaluating and offering feedback all increase the value of educational opportunities.

Introduction

This book is about how dentists can determine their educational needs and address them through the use of 'personal development plans'. But, surely, we've missed out a stage? Don't we need to establish first of all that there *is* a need to learn and that dentists are willing and able to engage in the process?

You may feel that such a need is obvious and therefore does not merit further discussion but, as a profession, dentistry is at a crossroads in many ways, not least with regard to how dentists equip themselves for the educational demands of the future. The knowledge, skills and attitudes required for the rest of our professional lives may not be the same as those that many dentists acquired as students and in the early days of practice life.

So it could be with education. Although the demands to analyse our work, show improvements in patient care and root out the 'bad apples' in our midst feel like an imposition, it is probably the greatest opportunity we have had to focus our learning on what *we* think matters. The encouragement to learn from and help each other could lead to a change in culture in which dentists and their teams work together to bring about improvements in service and, just as importantly, in job satisfaction.

Who is this book for?

So much for the rhetoric, but who is this book written for and how can it help you? The personal development plan (PDP) is central to our future continuing professional development (CPD) and in this book we will learn how the plan is written and implemented. We will also look at a variety of techniques that can help us to identify our needs and evaluate our progress.

The text could be read from cover to cover, but is probably better used as a learning resource that can be dipped into and out of according to need and interest. The book is written for generalists by generalists and is intended to be both credible and practical. To prove this point, before reading on, look at the examples of real PDPs on pages 67–79, which capture the spirit of the book.

We anticipate that the book will principally be read by general dental practitioners (GDPs) and it contains numerous *Checkpoints* represented by the symbol ☑ with questions and discussion to help readers test their understanding of the concepts involved. To obtain the maximum benefit these questions should be answered before the discussion is read.

The chapter on 'How to evaluate the PDP' (Chapter 5) will help dentists to improve the quality of their learning, but will prove particularly helpful to those in the teaching and training community.

Finally, the techniques that this book covers, such as significant event analysis, will gain greater prominence in the near future. The relevant chapters can be referred to when needed and will allow readers to become conversant with the hows as well as the whys of these approaches. These chapters will be particularly helpful if used as background reading material prior to group discussion with other dentists and the dental team.

In the first chapter we consider why our approach to CPD needs to change and how we can begin to achieve this.

Why does our CPD need to change?

When a newly graduated dentist is admitted to the dental register or when a dentist continues to register on an annual basis, there is a requirement that the practitioner keeps up to date with the latest developments in his chosen field, whether it be general or specialist practice. Furthermore and, perhaps, more importantly, there is public expectation that healthcare professions have processes in place to ensure that CPD is carried out and is quality assured.

The GDC (General Dental Council) Lifelong Learning Scheme has now formalised this for the purpose of recertification. The GDC scheme, which is now mandatory, requires dental practitioners to undertake 15 hours of verifiable CPD and another 35 hours of non-verifiable CPD each year during a five-year rolling cycle. In due course, a sample of dental practitioners, taken from a cohort of colleagues qualifying during a particular period, will be subject to scrutiny of their CPD records. If these are found to be deficient, the dentist will be given a period of grace in which to rectify the problem or risk being removed from the register.

Verifiable CPD is fairly easy to record as there is proof through the attendance register. However, non-verifiable CPD (often forgotten) may not appear so easy to log because it embraces aspects of learning and reflection that do not have tangible evidence of 'attendance'. This non-verifiable element could become the Cinderella of CPD because of the difficulty with producing appropriate evidence. However, it is in this very area that PDPs come into their own as they provide the mechanism to direct our learning to our needs and provide an appropriate record for the GDC scheme.

The GDC is now working on the next stage in the process of ensuring that dental practitioners are 'fit for purpose' – that is, competent to continue practising – by moving from recertification to revalidation. Revalidation is intended to ensure that we practise to the highest possible standard and provide the best quality of care for our patients and it will have CPD at its heart.

Of course, at first sight, all this appears to be quite threatening. However, apart from external forces that require the public to be protected (and remember we are all patients too), dentists have the self-motivation to continue to acquire new skills and to further develop themselves and their teams.

There is clearly then no better time to be innovative in the way we think about personal development. We need to move away from the philosophy of the perceived need (i.e. attending educational events that appear to support the things we like doing and to which many of us often go) and towards finding learning events that fit our personal 'needs assessment'. Clinical audit and peer review in the General Dental Service (GDS) are now a Terms of Conditions and Service requirement; in addition, it is likely that GDPs will be required to undergo some form of appraisal similar to that which hospital consultant colleagues are already undertaking.

Each of these forces – revalidation, appraisal and self-directed learning – will centre on the PDP and hence learning how to produce and implement one is both valuable and necessary.

How can we move on?

We have seen why our CPD needs to change. In this section we will first look at a model of how we learn, called the learning cycle, then use this as the basis from which to consider how improvements in our learning can take place.

The learning cycle (after Kolb)

This model demonstrates how experiences lead to a cycle of reflection and change which result in learning, as illustrated in Figure 1.1.

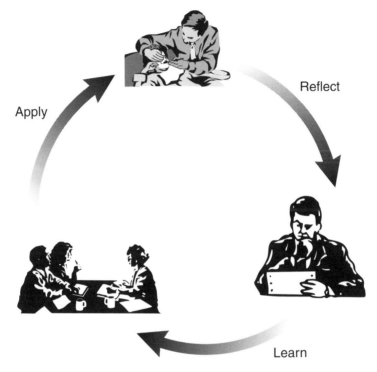

Figure 1.1 The learning cycle.

The dentist becomes aware that his inferior dental block is not working well, an *experience* which makes him uneasy and prompts him to *reflect* as to why this might be. This sense of unease alerts him to the fact that a gap exists between what he needs to know and what he actually knows. He realises that the cause of his discomfort is his lack of confidence about how best to give the injection and what to do when this fails. He therefore defines his *educational need* as learning how to improve his injection technique and learning a back-up technique that he can use when the block fails.

In order to *learn*, he has to identify not only what he needs to learn but also how he wishes to address that need, and on the basis of this he decides to do a literature search to identify best practice and to discuss the problem in a peer-review group. He finds that he is not alone in having difficulties but discovers that he can improve his technique by directing the barrel of the syringe towards the contralateral *upper* pre-molars, rather than the lower pre-molars. He also learns the intraligamentary injection technique to use as a back-up.

Having improved his skills, he is now able to *apply* his learning so that the next time he has to give the block, he feels good because he has more confidence in getting it right first time and he knows what to do if this fails.

Figure 1.1 indicates that thinking about such experiences, putting them into context and considering their implications (the process of reflecting) allows us to learn from them and decide whether changes are needed. Changes are not always welcomed, but if they are regarded as improvements that *we* wish to make, then they are more likely to be put into effect.

We will now look more closely at three elements in the learning cycle: experience, reflection and learning.

Using our experiences effectively

The first thing to recognise is that *experiences* are the raw material from which we define our learning needs. All experiences have this potential, even the seemingly trivial ones, and they are derived from:

- what we *do* – through assessing patients, carrying out procedures, etc.
- what we become *aware of* – through reading, feedback, complaints, audit and analysis of data, etc.
- what we *feel* – for example, in response to significant events in our practice lives.

Although we could learn from *all* experiences, in reality some experiences highlight more important learning needs than others, a point which is considered in Chapter 2.

Next, we need to raise our awareness so that we notice relevant experiences when they occur. Mostly, these experiences occur incidentally in our working lives and can therefore easily be lost unless they are recorded in a form such as a learning log.

In Chapter 6 on PUNs & DENs we look at the use of one such log which is derived from the contacts we have with patients.

Learning to reflect

Unfortunately, we often fail to recognise the importance of reflection as a key element of our professional development. Vocational dental practitioners were among the first dentists required to have a PDP. Experience has shown that rather than use reflection to identify their educational needs or to evaluate the success or otherwise of their learning, many simply completed their plans with a tick-box mentality. As Grieveson* has advised, we need to embrace the philosophy of reflective practice in order to achieve the potential of the PDP.

Once we recognise the need for reflective practice, we must develop the conditions in which it can occur. Thinking about our experiences allows us to reflect on those which make us feel uneasy and translate them into educational needs. This requires time which could be used more effectively if protected, and it is therefore useful to consider *when* we spend time reflecting. We recognise the importance of being free from distraction in our surgeries, where we seek to avoid having our work interrupted, but the concept is just as important for periods of reflection when our subconscious minds are busy working.

A factor not often considered is that reflection is aided by being in a suitable environment. Hence *where* we do our thinking is important and, if a suitable place does not already exist, it is worth finding or creating an environment in which we feel relaxed enough to think about the implications of our experiences. Environmental influences often work in a Pavlovian manner such that being in favoured surroundings quickly helps to get us into the right frame of mind.

Making the most of our learning opportunities

We will consider this by looking at three areas: how as colleagues we can help each other, how we learn best and how to get the best value from the educational events we attend.

---

* Grieveson B (2002) Assessment in dental vocational training: can we do better? *BDJ Educ Suppl.* **Sept.**

How can we help each other?

Learning together means admitting that we have things to learn, or in other words that we have 'failings'. How then does this make us feel and what could we do to encourage the process and ensure that the experience is a positive one for those who take part in it?

Initially this may involve cultivating a relationship with a colleague, talking about work experiences, as well as sharing ideas and opinions. Later, as barriers break down and people start to talk about their deficiencies, this may take the form of actively listening and encouraging without being directive. The temptation to tell colleagues how *we* would do things should be resisted, and instead they should be encouraged to express *their* thoughts, what they see the problems as being and what strategies they can think of to address them. Those people who are thought to offer wise advice in fact rarely tend to give answers but guide others to find their own.

What are the best ways of learning?

The purpose of postgraduate education is to bring about improvements (i.e. changes) in the way we work. Therefore, it is worth cultivating those forms of learning which have led to changes in practice. Additionally, careful thought should be given to time spent on educational activities which consistently reap little reward.

The following exercise can help to make the distinction.

☑ **Checkpoint 1.1**

Think about three improvements that you have made to your clinical practice in the past three years. Write down what these changes are and the educational activities which prompted you to change.

Now consider how representative these activities are of the way you currently learn and ask yourself whether you should be engaging in them more often. For example, attending a hands-on course might be much more likely to encourage change than learning about the same technique in a lecture.

We might well find that a proportion of the changes made were as a consequence of significant events in practice life. Recognising these as important influences for change might encourage us to use significant event analysis, as described in Chapter 7.

It is worth comparing our responses to this exercise with those of our colleagues. It may transpire that there are some forms of education that most people seem to gain benefit from and which could therefore be usefully encouraged. On this basis we might decide that clinical audit should be routinely conducted or that practice-based educational meetings offering the chance for discussion should be arranged.

What about the educational events that we attend?

Practice-based learning is becoming more important, because it relates directly to our particular needs. However, much external education will still be provided on behalf of dentists and there are steps that we can take to maximise the value of the events on offer.

These include the following.

- Attending events which address our needs and not attending those which don't.
- Playing an active part by contributing our perspective and insights, encouraging our colleagues to do likewise and questioning the relevance to dental practice. These factors help to keep such events focused and useful.
- Asking 'Will this change the way I think or practise?' rather than just 'Did I enjoy the meeting?', as this gives a better idea of whether the educational event was a good use of our time. Hopefully, the two are not incompatible!
- Giving appropriate feedback to the course organisers. Evaluation sheets are getting better, and could include the following questions.
  - Were the objectives of the event achieved?
  - What did you learn?
  - In what way will your practice change as a result?
  - If the event was to be repeated, in what way could it be improved?
  Even if the forms do not ask these questions, trying to answer them and offering responses to those running the meeting is very useful. Most of the steps taken above also apply to practice-based meetings, at which we could think about using evaluation forms for the reasons already mentioned.

Summary

Postgraduate dental education is now moving higher on the political agenda. The changes proposed will require dentists to think more carefully about what they are learning and why, and to work with other colleagues and team members in achieving common goals. Far from being threatening, this will offer an opportunity to make education both more relevant and more enjoyable, an aim that can be achieved through planning what needs to be learned and reflecting on how useful that learning has been. But before such plans can be made we need to identify where our deficiencies lie and decide how we wish to prioritise them. This is the subject of the next chapter.

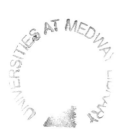

2 Identifying our learning needs

Introduction

Learning from our experiences

The methods of establishing our educational needs

Prioritising our learning needs

Summary

Key points

■ Our needs are derived from a wide range of sources.

■ Some sources are better suited to identifying particular needs than others.

■ It is preferable to be familiar with a variety of techniques for establishing our needs.

■ A number of agencies will have an influence on our educational priorities.

■ We therefore need to set our priorities in consultation with others.

■ A practical approach is to attend to safety first, then to national and local priorities.

■ Most priorities will still arise from our personal agenda.

Introduction

In the previous chapter, we established the importance of basing our education on needs rather than wants and of using our experiences to initiate learning cycles. In this chapter we will bring these themes together and consider where our experiences come from and how they can be used to identify deficiencies and therefore educational needs. Finally, we will consider the influences that make us prioritise certain needs and not others.

Learning from our experiences

Look at Figure 2.1, which has at its centre the learning cycle which was discussed in Chapter 1. The dentist treating the patient has an experience, in this case a sense of unease derived from giving a dental block, which leads on to a learning cycle. However, he could just as easily initiate learning cycles from other types of experiences drawn from the range of methods shown around him.

Each of these methods has the potential to make the dentist aware that he has a 'competence gap', which is a discrepancy between his current performance and the way he feels he would like to (or should) perform.

The methods of establishing our educational needs

Each of the methods shown in Figure 2.1 is discussed in more detail below. No one method is superior to the others, because in practice some methods are better suited to identifying certain needs compared with others. For instance, our communication skills with patients are probably better assessed through a suitable patient satisfaction questionnaire than by relying on our own impressions.

In addition, not all methods will be available or be suitable. Not all practices, for example, will have the facility to use computer-assisted learning, and very few practices are involved in research activity. Therefore to get a balance it is better not to rely on a single method, but to become familiar with the techniques that are feasible in the practice and use the appropriate ones according to the circumstances.

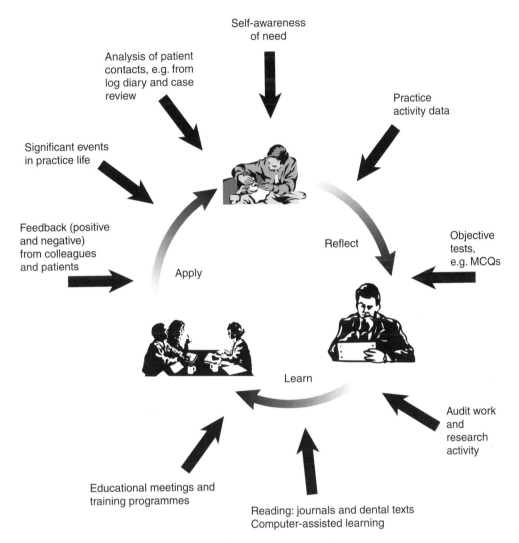

Figure 2.1 How dentists learn.

Self-awareness of need

Self-awareness, or using our opinion of our strengths and weaknesses in order to determine our educational needs, suffers from its lack of objectivity. Health professionals have been shown to be poor at correctly identifying their deficiencies, but provided that we do not rely upon this method alone and are honest with ourselves, self-awareness can be a powerful tool. Here are two exercises to help get self-awareness working for us.

☑ **Checkpoint 2.1**

- Imagine that you are in surgery and have just called your next patient. List the following:
  - the three types of problem with which you would feel most comfortable if presented
  - the three types of problem with which you would feel least comfortable if presented.
- Suppose that the time has come for the lines of responsibility within the practice to be redrawn and the dentists need to decide who among them is going to take a lead role with regard to important tasks such as business planning, nursing issues, team development and so on. List the following:
  - the three areas of responsibility with which you would feel most comfortable
  - the three areas of responsibility with which you would feel least comfortable.

Another approach is to ask:

- Which topics do I most enjoy learning about?
- Which topics do I least enjoy learning about?

Answering these questions with honesty allows us to reach more valid conclusions. Among the areas for which we have personal responsibility, we should think carefully about the ones that we find difficult and would prefer to avoid. Do these highlight educational needs, and if so do they need to be prioritised?

Significant events

Anything that is out of the ordinary in our personal or professional lives, and is significant either by its nature or because of its repercussions, is likely to be on our minds and has the potential to be learned from.

These events can often be powerful motivators for change in our professional behaviour. Mostly, change occurs when negative (or critical) events occur, but there are also lessons to be learned from positive events. The process of learning from these is called significant event analysis and is discussed in Chapter 7.

Feedback from colleagues and patients

This is a most important method of reviewing each other's work and making suggestions. Practices that do not meet either formally or informally (for example, in a coffee room) will miss out on what many dentists consider to be the most valuable method of learning. The quality of this experience can be improved by discussing various aspects of practice performance with local colleagues, either as a CPD group or as a peer-review group. Such discussion shows dentists how they compare with their colleagues, in a setting that is supportive rather than competitive.

Feedback from those we work with often comes in verbal form or from entries in patients' records, and some dentists gain additional feedback through more formal systems such as case review, clinical audit or the use of formal rating tools such as 360° feedback. The latter can provide feedback in an anonymised form on various areas beyond clinical performance, such as professional behaviour, team-working, communication and management, using the perspective of all those that we work with or for – hence 360°.

Patients may also provide feedback through avenues such as suggestions and complaints, by completing questionnaires or via patient participation groups.

Dentists do not manage their patients in isolation from their colleagues or indeed their patients, and feedback from them shows us what went well in addition to what might have been done better. Giving colleagues feedback on positive as well as negative events prevents a culture of blame developing, and it is important that when negative criticism *is* intended that it is delivered sensitively: 'Do as you would be done by' is a good approach.

No one enjoys being criticised and although feeling bad is a natural reaction and seems not to diminish with experience, ultimately there is satisfaction to be had in being honest with ourselves and in trying to improve where this is needed. When on the receiving end of criticism, after the initial flurry of denial has settled down, it is useful to ask ourselves whether, if faced with the same situation, we would act any differently. If the answer to this question is 'No', then either the criticism was not justified or our judgement is lacking. If the answer is 'Yes', then we have succeeded in identifying a learning need.

Analysis of clinical contacts

By this, we mean analysis of the records we keep following consultations with patients. These are rarely a full record of what went on in the consultation, but they can be examined to determine what we did, as well as what we didn't do and why. One approach, described in Chapter 6 on PUNs & DENs, is to look *prospectively* for our learning needs. After each patient contact, we briefly note whether the patient had an area of need of which we were aware but did not address. We can then use this insight to decide whether such unmet needs might be due to an educational deficiency on our part or not.

Another method is to look *retrospectively* at our records using the benefit of hindsight. We may be prompted to do this by a significant event or the feedback of another colleague involved in the patient's care. Suppose, for example, that a young adult is found to have gross caries. Following this we may decide to conduct a retrospective case review looking at the patient's notes and asking ourselves if appropriate assessments were performed and preventive care was given.

Sometimes there are guidelines or protocols which define good practice, such as the regulations for ionising radiation. Using these to audit our care, we can determine how aware we are of the recommendations, and to what degree they are being implemented.

Analysis of patient contact is a method that is frequently used in peer review, as dentists routinely review their work and compare it with that of their colleagues. Thus we may find that our amalgam fillings seem to fracture more frequently than those provided by our colleagues, which may lead us to think about the quality of our amalgam material and the adequacy of our cavity preparation technique.

Practice activity data

Looking at *practice activity data* means analysing the pattern of our tests, investigations and treatments along with the referrals that we make to colleagues inside and outside the practice. Through this, we can make comparisons of numbers and discuss why differences exist. For example, we might audit the periodontal pocket chartings of the dentists in the practice and look to see whether scores were improving with time. If they were not, this *might* indicate a lack of appropriate advice. On the practice management front, we might audit uncollected patient charges, which might reveal that certain colleagues were failing to advise patients appropriately about charges prior to treatment, thereby leading to complaints and a failure to pay. An audit on this topic is shown in Chapter 8 on page 174.

Objective tests

Because we direct our education to the problems we commonly encounter, although we may notice that our knowledge is developing in some areas we may not be aware that it is diminishing in others. It is said that our *confidence* in dealing with problems diminishes rather more slowly than our *competence* and many dentists recognise this to be true. To maintain competence as generalists we require an up-to-date knowledge of the basic areas of our subject, so how can we determine the areas in which our knowledge is lacking? Objective tests provide a mechanism for doing this and nowadays are tailored to practising dentists rather than just those taking exams, with their focus being on what we *need* to know rather than what we *could* know. A number also provide mini-tutorials and some of the best are available as computer-assisted learning (CAL) packages on CD-ROMs or the Internet.

Examples of these include:

- *The Dental Management of the Medically Compromised Patient*, produced by Eastman Dental Institute
- *Aspects of Partial Denture Design*, by John Davenport.

In addition, there are numerous well-known endodontic CAL disks that many GDPs now use. CAL programs are often available through the deaneries. As an example, *see* www.pgde-trent.co.uk.

Educational meetings

Meetings are extremely popular and provide an opportunity both to learn and to network with our colleagues. It is said, probably correctly, that most of the learning in many meetings and conferences occurs not during the lecture but in the coffee break!

Traditionally, most meetings for GDPs are given by consultants and academics and the assumption is that secondary care sets the gold standard against which GDPs should measure themselves and to which they should aspire. However, generalists are not mini-specialists but are experts in the field of general dental practice. This means that the educational impact of many meetings could be improved by framing the tuition in a generalist context. Even better, GDPs could be involved in developing the educational objectives for the meeting and chairing the meeting to ensure that a generalist focus is maintained.

All lectures can be improved by allowing sufficient time for feedback, questioning and discussion, especially if groups are kept small to facilitate the contribution of individuals.

It is preferable to attend meetings not simply out of interest, but because we think that we might learn something. During the meeting, we should be on the lookout for those times when we feel uneasy with the subject material as these points might signify the presence of competence gaps which need addressing. Because meetings are quickly forgotten, it is best to make a note of these gaps as soon after the meeting as possible.

The meeting should have some learning objectives specified by the organiser, and at the end of the meeting we should decide to what extent these objectives have been met. We might do this, for example, by completing a formal evaluation form such as that shown on pages 114–15. If they were *not* met, we should consider whether the fault lay with the presenter or with ourselves.

Audit work and research activity

Dentists are funded to undertake only a limited number of hours of either peer review or audit activity over a three-year period. Unsurprisingly, peer review wins hands down because of the fact that it is more sociable and does not require much preparatory work.

However, audit is the most powerful way of identifying our gaps. Because it is a method of measuring our performance against certain standards, audit can both identify these gaps and indicate how large they are. The audit standards may be set by ourselves but occasionally national standards may be available. Audit encourages objectivity and, by showing how far short we fall of the standard, audit can help us to decide how urgently we need to address the area under scrutiny. Finally, by completing the audit cycle we can objectively measure our success at learning and at changing our practice. The mechanism and potential of clinical audit are discussed in Chapter 8.

Research provides the evidence-base for our work and is increasingly being performed within the community, which increases its applicability to general dental practice. Dentists can learn much by engaging in this research, either by providing data for research projects or by conducting research of their own.

Reading

Certain forms of learning are better gained through reading than by attending lectures. For example, if we wished to improve our understanding of the theory of how nickel-titanium files prepare the root canal for obturation, we would need to look at appropriate diagrams in the endodontic journals.

Such journals, dental textbooks and, more recently, Internet sources provide the basis for keeping up to date. The problem lies with prioritising the vast array of information which is available to us and there is a need to triage the literature in order to decide first what to read and second whether to act on it. To learn how to prioritise journals and articles, it is worth reading the article by MaCauley (1994) *Br J Gen Pract* **44**: 83–5 in which the READER acronym is described. This system ascribes scores to articles on the basis of their:

- Relevance to general dental practice
- Educational value in bringing about a change in behaviour
- Applicability to our own practice
- Discrimination in terms of methodology.

We can't change our practice in the light of *all* new developments, so deciding what we should take notice of, and what we should ignore, enables us to make our learning effective.

Appraisal

Appraisal is a supportive and formative process designed to help all health professionals to develop their professional skills through consideration of their educational needs and resource requirements and has an explicit link to the PDP. Chapter 9 explains the process in more detail.

Being an exercise that encourages reflection on learning and career development, appraisal may alter a dentist's priorities for the coming year.

For example, suppose that our initial perceptions indicated a personal deficiency in orthodontics, brought to light because this was done by an associate who left the practice.

Discussion in the appraisal meeting might suggest that this was not in fact an educational priority because we had neither the interest to develop the orthodontic skills nor the time and resources required to complete the higher training course that would be required to meet this need. We might decide that it would be better to refer our patients to the dental hospital or to employ a suitably qualified associate.

Conversely, an educational need might be added as a result of the appraisal process. For example, time and stress management may not be perceived as being a problem in practitioners who feel that they are coping well. However, an opportunity to talk these issues through with time for reflection may disclose that the pressures are still there, not too deeply buried beneath the surface. A need to learn how to handle stress and prevent burnout might thereby be identified.

Prioritising our learning needs

Using the range of methods discussed, we may gain many experiences from which our educational needs can be identified. Once these needs have been recognised, we need to prioritise *which* of them we propose attending to and *in what order*. Our decision will be influenced by personal needs, the needs of the practice, external agencies and the pressure of time, as depicted in Figure 2.2.

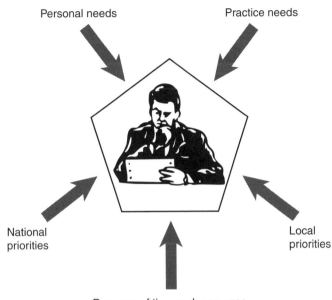

Personal needs

Practice needs

National priorities

Local priorities

Pressure of time and resources

Figure 2.2 Prioritising our needs: the influences on GDPs.

Because the priorities which are set are influenced by other agencies, it is better if we can decide on them in consultation with our colleagues. Although there are no rules with regard to deciding which educational needs should be attended to first, the following represents a practical approach.

Safety first

Potentially, there is a tension between the desires of the individual and the wishes of others regarding which needs are prioritised, because individuals will want to retain ownership of their educational activity. However, most parties would agree that safety and basic competence are the first priority.

Therefore when we look at our educational needs, we have to ask: 'What are the implications for patient care of *not* prioritising this need?', and the more serious the consequences for the patient, the more urgently should the need be addressed. Hence, if we were involved in a significant event such as the inhalation of a dental file during root canal treatment, we would urgently need to consider using rubber dam routinely.

Obeying orders

Increasingly, there are directives from other bodies that have to be carried through at practice level. For example, the Department of Health requires us to secure the oral health of patients receiving NHS treatment, which would require us to routinely use basic periodontal evaluation (BPE) charting at recall visits. Guidelines from organisations such as the National Institute for Clinical Excellence (NICE) recommend how certain conditions should be managed across the nation. Likewise, paymasters such as the Dental Practice Board require evidence of radiographs prior to bridge work or crowns. We need to ensure that we have the skills to carry these directives through and if we have educational needs that fall within the topic areas, then these should be given priority.

Practice development

Once the wider expectations are met, we are free to attend to the other needs of our practice. The practice development plan (or business plan) will set goals that require particular skills from the team members and we may therefore decide to tailor part of our educational programme to meet these requirements. For example, if patients were increasingly requesting aesthetic treatment, we might decide to learn how to bleach teeth or place new materials such as ceramic inlays and onlays, thus expanding our services and increasing practice income.

Personal agenda

Although seemingly at the bottom of the list, most of the priorities we set from our list of educational needs will arise from our personal agenda, but how we choose the priorities requires consideration. A good place to start is to think about those deficiencies which cause us the greatest unease. These quite often arise from significant events, even those that don't have the risk of patient harm. Correcting these deficiencies helps us not only in educational terms but also in being able to put the event behind us and move on at a personal level.

It is also useful to think of any longer-term plans that we have for our professional development as these goals might dictate the skills that we need to acquire. For example, we may have ambitions regarding vocational training and may therefore wish to go on a course for potential trainers.

Our personal needs may relate to our everyday work. For example, we may wish to learn about the alternative techniques for the provision of complete replacement dentures, such as the replica or copy techniques. Alternatively, repeated experience with anxious patients may encourage us to think about learning how to use inhalational or intravenous sedation techniques.

Many needs relating to dental practice are not simply clinical. As an example, the higher levels of computer literacy which are becoming mandatory for all clinicians, including dentists, may encourage us to develop our skills in this area.

Summary

The experiences from which dentists can learn are all around us and are part of the fabric of our working lives. In this chapter we have looked at the sources of these experiences, some of which will be familiar but others may offer new routes for learning. Four of these sources, namely PUNs & DENs, significant event analysis, clinical audit and appraisal, are particularly fruitful and will be considered in detail in Chapters 6–9.

Identifying and prioritising our educational needs ensures that the limited time we have to attend to these needs is optimally spent, and in the next chapter we will discuss how we can take an educational need and address it through the use of a personal development plan.

3 Personal development plans: an overview

Key points

- PDPs (personal development plans) are a mechanism by which we prioritise our educational needs and make a commitment to attend to them.
- They also demonstrate to outsiders that we have a professional approach to our CPD.
- The evidence that we collect for our PDP will prove useful for revalidation.
- The plans are owned by ourselves, although we should take account of the needs of our practice.
- Each plan is written for a year, but is part of an upward spiral of professional development.
- Currently, we may attend courses because they are available and we may verify our learning by collecting certificates of attendance.

- PDPs change the emphasis by encouraging us to be proactive.
- They help us to direct our learning appropriately and to reflect on its usefulness to our professional development.

Introduction

Society has changed and one manifestation of this is the change in the way that professionals are perceived by the public. If we regarded this in a negative light, we might bemoan the loss of autonomy and the 'interference' by those who don't seem to understand the discipline or appreciate the high standards that dentists set for themselves. Unfortunately, self-regulation doesn't always protect the public, as several high-profile cases have shown and health professionals are adjusting to the fact that even though they are likely be perfectly competent, they must be *seen* to be so.

In relation to postgraduate education, dentists will not be assumed to be up to date but will need to demonstrate their competence by providing appropriate information relating to the fields in which they practise. Current methods of continuing dental education involve attending meetings, sitting (or dozing) through lectures and collecting accreditation forms. This approach is problematic as it does not accredit the time that we spend learning in practice, may result in loss of earnings and is often ineffective at producing change. This is where the PDP comes in, both as a mechanism by which we can demonstrate to others that we have a systematic approach to our education and as a method for making our learning more effective. Seen in this way, there is a silver lining of educational benefit to the cloud of public expectation.

In this chapter, we will learn about the PDP process, look at the paperwork involved and see it illustrated through an example. In Chapter 4, a simple approach will be demonstrated by which to write the first PDP, and in Chapter 5, the principles that allow us to evaluate the PDP will be discussed in detail.

Note: if you prefer not to read too much detail initially, you may wish to read Chapter 4 at this point, which is only a few pages long, and then return to this chapter.

What is a PDP?

Quite simply, the PDP is a process by which we identify our educational needs, set ourselves some objectives in relation to these, undertake our educational activities and produce evidence that we have learned something useful.

☑ **Checkpoint 3.1**

Each of the three words 'personal', 'development' and 'plan' has significance. Because the PDP is the cornerstone of professional development, it is important that you make your own interpretation of the purpose and potential of the plan. You can do this by answering the following questions in relation to the key words.

- *Personal*: how personal should the plan be? Should it relate to your own needs or should it be broader?

- *Development*: what does 'development' mean? In your view, what aspects of your professional development should the plan address?

- *Plan*: what are the implications of having a plan? How long a period should the plan cover?

☑ **Checkpoint 3.1 discussion**

There are no right or wrong answers to the questions posed. Rather, there is a range of perspectives and the following comments are drawn from the experience of dental educators.

- *Personal*: there are many (and increasing) influences on our professional practice. New requirements like clinical audit and clinical governance raise expectations that dentists will prioritise certain areas of clinical practice for closer scrutiny and thereby for further education. Although these areas may be identified through consensus with fellow colleagues, they may not reflect the dentist's personal needs. Therefore, it would seem sensible to keep the emphasis of the

PDP on the learner because the PDP is the main vehicle by which personal needs can be legitimately prioritised. Of course, this does not mean that the PDP should bear no relation to the context of a dentist's work. For instance, the circumstances of a dentist's practice, such as the skill mix and the dental health of the population, would quite naturally influence the skills that the dentist needs and therefore his development plan.

- *Development*: the word implies progression or a positive change from the status quo and this means that the plan should indicate both the current position and the desired goal. 'Development' should be viewed broadly as encompassing not just the obvious clinical needs but also other areas of professional life in which further education is required to achieve a particular goal. For example, it would be quite legitimate for a dentist who felt disadvantaged through not being computer literate to include basic IT skills, such as learning to use email or producing a Word document, in his plan. Likewise, a dentist with training responsibilities might wish to learn how to facilitate problem-based learning and might therefore incorporate this in his PDP.

- *Plan*: the fact that the PDP is a *plan* represents a major difference between the PDP and other systems of recording CPD activity. As we will see later, the PDP is written at the start of the year and the learner is encouraged to identify a few needs and then plan how they might be implemented. In other words, the process of learning is proactive rather than reactive.

This does not mean that experiential learning is in any way second-best. Learning in response to the events of daily life is vital but depends by definition on what is encountered and is therefore subject to chance. A development plan offers us the opportunity to decide what we need to learn about and then to plan how to meet this need. A further implication of having a plan is that it creates in us a sense of commitment that we will see the plan through.

The plan usually covers a one-year period, meaning that the educational needs that we commit ourselves to meeting should be completed within this timescale. However, this should not be seen as restricting our ability to plan for the longer term. There are many important needs, e.g. training for a postgraduate diploma, that take much longer than a year to complete and these can be incorporated in the PDP by selecting learning needs from the diploma in each successive year. Having a timescale is important as, without it, our back burner just gets overloaded!

Common questions

Now that we have established what a plan is, let us consider how to write the plan by answering the following.

☑ **Checkpoint 3.2**

- Who should write the PDP? Should it be the learner alone or should others be involved?
- What should we put in the PDP? Should we include everything that we learn?
- How many learning needs should we aim to meet in any given year?
- How do we know if our plan is good enough? Who writes the rules?

☑ **Checkpoint 3.2 discussion**

Writing the PDP
The PDP is owned by the learner, who has principal responsibility for writing the plan. However, it is often helpful to write the plan in conjunction with our colleagues, usually our partners in the practice. The advantages are as follows.

- Practices increasingly look to formulate a *practice development plan* covering periods of one or more years. This plan may contain business and managerial goals, but will often have clinical implications that may influence the educational needs of the dentists. The requirement to undertake clinical audit will also need to be taken into account and these factors can legitimately and usefully influence the contents of each learner's PDP.

- No one wants to do the same work twice. If the practice requires us to develop our skills in a particular area and we are also required to have a PDP, then why not combine the two? This is not 'cheating', as the purpose of ongoing dental education is to produce benefits for our patients, and therefore linking our personal agenda with that of the practice is a vital way of creating these benefits.

- If the practice collectively decides upon certain goals and identifies the associated educational needs, it usually shares responsibility for meeting those needs. In some practices this may mean financial help but, even if not, collective responsibility means mutual support, encouragement and help with time-out for education.

- Writing the PDP requires us to decide where our deficiencies lie, what our specific objectives are and what evidence we might keep for our portfolio to show that we have learned something. Each of these elements can be much more easily determined through discussion with a colleague and many dentists find that small-group discussion is both productive and helps to augment professional relationships.

The contents of the PDP
- The PDP is not intended to be a comprehensive record of *everything* that we learn. Most of our learning occurs in the normal course of our working days through our practical experiences with patients, discussion with colleagues and through our reading. This learning is often small scale, but it is frequent and the incremental effect over time is significant.

- The hours that we spend learning may amount to several hundred during the course of the year and it would be an impossible (and unhelpful) task to attempt to record this!

- External agencies require us to demonstrate that we have a systematic approach to our CPD and the PDP is simply the tip of our learning iceberg. However, it is the part that we choose to present for this purpose.

The number of learning needs
- For professionals in other spheres, e.g. doctors and nurses, the PDP is used to demonstrate that a set number of approved hours of educational activity have been undertaken per annum. In a similar way, it is possible that we could qualify for our non-verifiable hours of CPD activity through undertaking a PDP.

- As the PDP only requires us to demonstrate a limited number of hours of educational activity, the number of learning needs does not have to be large and the exact number will depend on how time-consuming each one is to fulfil.

- For example, learning how to decide whether a white patch in the mouth should be referred may simply be a matter of reading a textbook. On the other hand, learning how to perform implant surgery will involve many hours in attending a course and gaining hands-on experience.

- On average, attending to around three needs per annum seems appropriate and feasible.

The guidelines
- Plans should not be thought of as being 'good' or 'bad' on the basis of the learning needs that the dentist wishes to address. Every practitioner has different strengths and weaknesses and works in different circumstances. Additionally, dentists vary in their ability to recognise their weaknesses and in their willingness to admit to them and take action. Seemingly straightforward needs might surprise some colleagues but may be a sign of honesty and, in that context, should be applauded.

- However, we can criticise the *structure* of a PDP because plans that are very unfocused, with no specific objectives or ideas as to how the educational needs might be met, are less likely to help the learner to achieve his aim and can therefore be said to be 'bad'.

- There are no national rules governing the process of personal development planning or of the contents of the PDP. However, this does not mean that no guidelines exist. PDPs may be required by outsiders but their principal purpose is to help the learner to develop professionally. Plans vary in their ability to help the learner to achieve this aim and, in Chapter 5, we will use many examples of PDPs to see how to make our plans as effective as possible.

The PDP spiral

Although we have defined the PDP as a one-year plan, it should not be thought of as a written plan in isolation, but as part of a process. Let us imagine that we are starting from scratch, in which case the process is as illustrated in Figure 3.1.

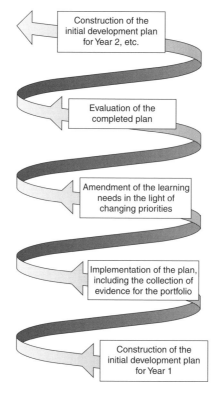

Figure 3.1 The PDP spiral.

I use the word 'spiral' rather than 'cycle' to emphasise that with every step, we are further on in our educational development than we were at the same time in the preceding year. This is a crucial point because, as we will see later, our completed development plan should be able to demonstrate educational *progress*, particularly with regard to improvements in patient care.

To get a feel for the PDP spiral, let us look at each of the elements in more detail.

Construction of the initial development plan for Year 1

This involves sitting down and writing a plan that comprises a short list of perhaps one or two educational needs. Each of these needs is then sketched out in terms of how it might be met and what evidence might be kept for the portfolio to prove that we have undertaken the planned learning. An example of this is shown in Table 3.1.

Further examples from the real world can be found on pages 67–79.

Implementation of the plan, including the collection of evidence for the portfolio

Work can begin straight away on attending to our stated priorities. By implementation, we mean undertaking the learning activities that we have decided to use, be they reading, being taught a new skill on a course and so on. Because circumstances change, we do not have to stick to the methods stated in our initial plan and we may find that other activities become available that prove to be more appropriate. For example, the availability of a computer-assisted learning (CAL) program may mean that we do not have to attend a course.

Whatever activities we ultimately use, they will give rise to some documentary proof of learning such as our written evaluation of them, and this paperwork may be used as evidence to be kept in our portfolio.

Amendment of the learning needs in the light of changing priorities

During the year, priorities will change. For instance, a learning need such as a radiography update may prove difficult to meet because the course is overbooked, or a new practice priority may result in our educational needs

Table 3.1: Initial development plan: orthodontics

Educational need	Reason for inclusion in development plan	Learning objectives	Activities to be used	What evidence will you keep?
To provide more orthodontic treatments for patients in the practice.	I use simple removable appliance orthodontics for a few patients, but don't feel confident to do more. Patients have long waiting times to see the specialist. I also wish to develop another clinical skill, and thereby maintain my interest and enthusiasm for daily general dental practice.	To be able to undertake fixed appliance treatment in my practice.	Clinical assistantship in orthodontics at the hospital. Literature search. Join the two-year part-time GP postgraduate practical fixed appliance course.	Literature résumés. Case review. Audit of practice appointment book: are more fixed appliances being provided?

being redefined. Amendments are therefore not only 'allowed' but they are inevitable and necessary.

Evaluation of the completed plan

Many people consider evaluation to be an essential part of the PDP process as through it dentists can learn valuable lessons from the success or otherwise of their development plan. This allows future learning to be better targeted and pitfalls that have led to failure in meeting the objectives to be avoided. Evaluation is done by the individual, but we can gain a great deal by discussing the outcomes of learning with a group of our colleagues.

Construction of the initial development plan for Year 2

Leading on from the evaluation, we can begin to plan the following year's plan whilst learning the lessons from the previous one.

Finally, evidence of learning which arises through implementing each year's PDP cycle can be collected in the portfolio and, if required, submitted every five years as part of revalidation, as shown in Figure 3.2.

Paperwork

In terms of bureaucracy, nothing could be simpler than the current system of turning up to a meeting, signing the register and collecting a certificate of attendance. Unfortunately, this system does not provide evidence that we have planned and evaluated our learning. Hence to write a PDP and complete the learning cycle, different paperwork is needed. The format shown below is that used by health professionals in the South Yorkshire and East Midlands area and has the advantage of maximising the educational benefits of PDPs while keeping the amount of writing required to a minimum.

Forms

These four sheets reflect each stage of the PDP cycle previously described, and comprise:

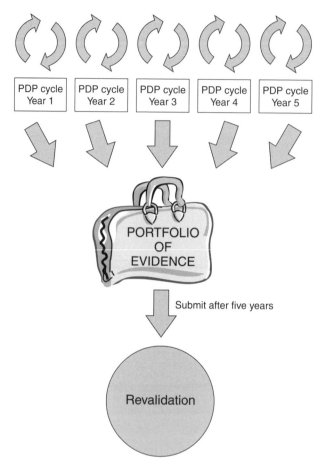

Figure 3.2 The link with revalidation.

- initial development plan
- amendment sheet
- activity summary
- evaluation.

The forms will now be described in more detail.

Initial development plan

This is written at the beginning of the year and is based on the dentists' perception of their educational priorities and which ones they wish to prioritise and commit themselves to meeting (*see* Table 3.2).

Table 3.2: Development plan: initial version

Educational need	Reason for inclusion in development plan	Learning objectives	Activities to be used	What evidence will you keep?
What is the general area in which you need to learn?	What has motivated you to prioritise this need?	Specifically, what knowledge or ability are you hoping to gain?	What methods might you use to obtain this?	What physical evidence will you keep for your portfolio to demonstrate what you have learned?

Table 3.3: Development plan: amendments

Educational need	Reason for including/ removing from development plan	Learning objectives for additions	Activities to be used for additions	What evidence will you keep?
What is the general area in which you need to learn?	What has motivated you to prioritise this need? *Or* Why is the learning need no longer a priority?	Specifically, what knowledge or ability are you hoping to gain?	What methods might you use to obtain this?	What physical evidence will you keep for your portfolio to demonstrate what you have learned?

Amendment sheet

Plans change, and every learner has the right to alter his initial plan in the light of circumstances and changing priorities. However, it is important that the learner thinks carefully about why changes are being made and the amendment form encourages this process (*see* Table 3.3).

Activity summary

Each educational need will usually be broken down into a small number of specific learning objectives that can be met by undertaking certain learning activities. We have noted that the initial learning plan merely identifies activities that *could* be used and evidence that *could* be kept. Because the evidence that is kept depends upon the activities that are undertaken, a change in the activities may lead to changes in the evidence. The activity summary is therefore a record of the *actual* activities undertaken and the actual evidence that was kept. In addition, this summary provides a log of the number of hours spent in educational activity – information that is needed if the PDP is being accredited for CPD purposes.

Table 3.4: Development plan: activity summary

Learning objective	Educational activities	What evidence have you kept?	Number of hours
The learning objective is stated here.	The actual activities used are listed.	The physical evidence of learning is stated.	The number of hours spent on learning in relation to this objective is stated.

Evaluation

The guiding principle behind personal development plans is that dentists should be encouraged to be 'adult learners', setting and meeting their own educational challenges. We have seen how PDPs require us to think carefully about our learning needs before we make a start. At the end of the year, the usual inclination would be to collect the evidence and cross the PDP off the 'to do' list. However, there is much to be gained by putting time aside to reflect upon the usefulness of the PDP and, to allow for this, the last of the PDP forms encourages us to undertake self-evaluation. A brief explanation of the questions is given below and the purpose of asking them is discussed in Chapter 5.

Development plan: evaluation

How did you identify your learning needs for this PDP, and what other methods might you include in your next PDP?

Which technique did you use to decide what you need to learn, e.g. self-reflection, audit, etc.?

Which objectives were easiest to achieve and why?

Learning needs are broken down into objectives. Which of these did you find straightforward/quick to achieve? What was it about the objective that made it achievable?

Which objectives were most difficult to achieve and why?

Were there any objectives that you did *not* meet? If so, what were the barriers? Similarly, if objectives were arduous, what were the reasons?

Which were the most valuable learning activities and why?

Activities include reading, using the computer, peer review and going on courses. Which did you find that you learned the most from?

Which were the least valuable learning activities and why?

Alternatively, even if activities were enjoyable, you may not have learned much from them. Which were these, and why were they educationally unsuccessful?

In what ways have you been able to apply your learning in practice?

Having completed your plan, you may have gained knowledge, skills or new attitudes. Have you been able to apply any of these to your practice?

What benefits to your patients do you feel have occurred as a result of your learning?

If you have applied your learning, then some changes will have occurred in the way you work. Do you feel that any of these changes have resulted in direct improvements in patient care? If so, try to say what they are.

Which, if any, learning needs do you wish to carry forward to your next PDP?

Some needs may not have been met at all or to the degree that you had stated in your plan. If so, do you wish to move on to something new or do you feel that the unmet need should be attended to in next year's plan?

What does a completed plan look like?

Now that we have studied the paperwork, we can gain a better understanding of how to complete the forms by looking at Table 3.5.

Table 3.5: Development plan: initial version

Educational need	Reason for inclusion in development plan	Learning objectives	Activities to be used	What evidence will you keep?
Antibiotic prophylaxis.	I don't feel confident about the conditions for which I should be recommending prophylaxis against infective endocarditis.	1 Know which conditions are important. 2 Know which antibiotic regimes to recommend. 3 Know how to alert the dentist of the need for prophylaxis.	1 Reading. 2 Talk with partners and manager about disease register/record keeping/use of computer prompts.	Audit patients with predisposing conditions for infective endocarditis: have they received appropriate treatment?

☑ **Checkpoint 3.3**

Having read this initial plan, written at the start of the educational year, answer the following questions.

- What are your feelings about this dentist's stated educational need and his reason for prioritising it?
- How 'good' are the learning objectives?
- What do you think about the activities that are proposed – are they appropriate?
- Is the evidence suitable?
- What other evidence could have been chosen?

☑ **Checkpoint 3.3 discussion**

Educational needs and priorities
It could be said that no educational need is inappropriate if it is attending to a dentist's perceived deficiency. This dentist has identified what may seem to some as being a basic area of clinical knowledge. Basic areas are also fundamental and, on this basis alone, it would seem appropriate to prioritise it. Where several needs are identified, discussion with colleagues can help dentists to decide which needs to tackle first and this may be guided by the need to ensure patient safety, to help to meet practice objectives or to achieve personal goals.

In the second box the dentist stated his reason for tackling this need, which in this case is a lack of confidence in his knowledge. This is like an 'honesty box' and completing it helps us to check whether the learning need really *is* a priority – in other words, that it is something important in terms of patient care or personal development. It also helps us to gauge our motivation. The PDP comprises a number of learning needs that we claim to be committed to meeting. Because this commitment has resource implications in terms of time, effort and money, it is important that we check that we are sufficiently motivated to take action.

'Good' objectives
The purpose of objectives is to define the knowledge or abilities that we intend to gain through our education. They should be specific enough to allow us to tell when they have been achieved and should be feasible enough for us to be confident of success.

Suppose this dentist had written as his learning objective: 'Feel more confident about antibiotic prophylaxis.' Would this have met the criteria mentioned above? If we compare this to the objectives that he actually wrote, we should find that the latter are better because they are specific and therefore more likely to lead to success.

Activities
These appear straightforward and sensible. Reading would be a good method to meet the first two objectives and the proposed meetings could well help the learner to develop a system for attending to the third objective. Other common activities such as going to courses would not seem appropriate in this situation, but peer review, in which the dentist talked to neighbouring colleagues about their own systems and standards for identifying 'at-risk' patients, is likely to be useful.

Evidence
Producing evidence of learning rather than purely evidence of attendance is a new development in CPD and is not intuitive for most learners. As a guiding principle, it is best not to collect evidence that is useless to the learner and is only being produced because it is required for the purposes of accountability. The best evidence comprises documentation that the dentist would have wanted to produce for his own benefit. In the example shown, a clinical audit is a good way of showing not only application of learning but (hopefully) of improvement in practice. In addition, it would kill two birds with one stone as it would demonstrate involvement in audit, which is now a service requirement for dentists.

Audit is time-consuming and is not the only form of evidence that could be produced. Other examples might include a summary of the indications for antibiotic prophylaxis or a new management protocol written to address the third objective of providing a system to forewarn dentists that the patient requires antibiotic cover.

Table 3.6: Development plan: activity summary

Learning objective	Educational activities	What evidence have you kept?	Number of hours
Know how to alert the dentist of the need for prophylaxis.	1 Produced an action plan with the practice manager.	Action plan	0.75
	2 Discussed how to develop and maintain a disease register. Local medics very helpful, as always!	Meeting notes	1.0
	3 Learned how to link a computer prompt with disease register.	Protocol	1.0
	4 Discussed and agreed new protocol with partners.		0.5

This dentist went on to implement his development plan, and for each of his three objectives, he produced an activity summary. Table 3.6 relates to the third objective.

☑ **Checkpoint 3.4**

The activity summary provides a record of what was actually done and what evidence was kept, along with a log of the time spent. What are your thoughts about the following.

- Were the activities appropriate?
- Was the evidence appropriate and useful?
- Does the time taken seem reasonable?

☑ **Checkpoint 3.4 discussion**

Activities
These were well focused and seem appropriate. The dentist appears to have talked to several people, including the local dentists, and this wide discussion would be more likely to make the final protocol evidence-based and feasible.

Evidence
It is not necessary for every activity to give rise to evidence for the portfolio and it would have been quite reasonable for the learner to produce less evidence than he did. Ideally, evidence should indicate what the dentist has learned or how the learning has been applied. The action plan and protocol will have met these criteria, but the meeting notes may not have done if they were simply minutes.

In terms of the usefulness of evidence to the learner, it is possible that the dentist would not normally have kept notes following the meeting, but might have produced an action plan or protocol for his own benefit. Either of these would have been excellent evidence and would have been sufficient for the plan.

Number of hours
A common concern of learners is that they need to include many learning objectives in order to achieve the required number of hours of accredited

educational activity. As this example demonstrates, the hours accrue very quickly and therefore a large number of objectives is not needed.

For this learning objective alone, the learner engaged in over three hours of activity and the time claimed seems reasonable and may even be an underestimate. We know from experience that there can be few occasions on which agreement from the partners regarding a protocol can be gained in half an hour!

Having undertaken the plan, the learner has the opportunity to reflect on the work that he has done and how effective he has been. Look at the following evaluation.

Development plan: evaluation

How did you identify your learning needs for this PDP, and what other methods might you include in your next PDP?

Mostly by self-reflection. I did an audit to confirm that I was using antibiotics appropriately, and the audit technique is one that I could use next year to determine where my needs lie.

Which objectives were easiest to achieve and why?

Learning about the indications for antibiotics – just a matter of looking it up in a book.

Which objectives were most difficult to achieve and why?

Sorting out how I could make use of the computer to prompt me in surgery, because lots of other people were involved and I didn't feel confident about using the computer.

Which were the most valuable learning activities and why?

Talking with the practice manager about how to use the practice computer. She was patient with me and I felt a sense of achievement at being able to do more than just switch it on.

Which were the least valuable learning activities and why?

Discussing the protocol with the partners. Not everyone was enthusiastic and they were concerned that setting up the disease register was expensive and unnecessary.

In what ways have you been able to apply your learning to practice?

I've been alerted when antibiotic was needed at a time in advance of the consultation when appropriate advice could be given.

What benefits to your patients do you feel have occurred as a result of your learning?

Wasted consultations have been avoided and patients have been properly protected when they have attended for treatment such as scale and polish.

They have also commented favourably on our system which they say makes the practice seem more 'up to date'.

☑ **Checkpoint 3.5**

We will look at this evaluation in more detail in Chapter 5. At this point, what do you feel the learner may have gained overall from completing this form?

☑ **Checkpoint 3.5 discussion**

Up to this point, the learner has shown that he is capable of producing specific objectives that have increased the chance of success in meeting his educational needs. He has also undertaken appropriate activities and collected evidence that has shown that the plan has been implemented. However, implementation does not in itself guarantee that the outcomes of the plan will be reflected on and learned from. Without completing the self-evaluation, the learner may not have realised the following:

- the difficulty in fulfilling objectives when several people are needed to achieve success
- the value of learning from a colleague within the practice – in this case, the practice manager
- his personal feelings about computers
- the improvement not only in the service but in the patients' perception of the practice.

Evaluations of this sort help us in two ways. First, they encourage us to reflect on the *content* of our learning and decide whether attending to the needs that we have selected has resulted in any useful change to our practice. Second, they make us think about the *process* of learning with regard to the way that we learn and help us to gauge how successful our methods are.

Summary

The PDP is a simple concept but has fundamental implications for the way we learn. Experiential learning, i.e. learning on the job, will always be the bedrock of professional development and PDPs are not intended to replace this but rather to add a new dimension to our learning. Using this tool, we have the opportunity to be proactive and attend to what we need to learn rather than just go to courses that are selected simply because they are available. Having seen an example, in the next chapter we will look at the nuts and bolts of writing our first plan.

Development plan: initial version

Educational need	Reason for inclusion in development plan	Learning objectives	Activities to be used	What evidence will you keep?
What is the general area in which you need to learn?	What has motivated you to prioritise this need?	Specifically, what knowledge or ability are you hoping to gain?	What methods might you use to obtain this?	What physical evidence will you keep for your portfolio to demonstrate what you have learned?

Development plan: amendments

Educational need	Reason for including/ removing from development plan	Learning objectives for additions	Activities to be used for additions	What evidence will you keep?
What is the general area in which you need to learn?	What has motivated you to prioritise this need? Or Why is the learning need no longer a priority?	Specifically, what knowledge or ability are you hoping to gain?	What methods might you use to obtain this?	What physical evidence will you keep for your portfolio to demonstrate what you have learned?

Development plan: activity summary

Learning objective	Educational activities	What evidence have you kept?	Number of hours

Development plan: evaluation

How did you identify your learning needs for this PDP, and what other methods might you include in your next PDP?

Which objectives were easiest to achieve and why?

Which objectives were most difficult to achieve and why?

Which were the most valuable learning activities and why?

Which were the least valuable learning activities and why?

In what ways have you been able to apply your learning in practice?

What benefits to your patients do you feel have occurred as a result of your learning?

Which, if any, learning needs do you wish to carry forward to your next PDP?

4 PDPs: making a start

Key points

- ■ We must learn to walk before attempting to run. A basic PDP is easy to write – anyone can do it.
- ■ We need to keep our learning aims simple. The most important thing is to make a start.
- ■ It is better to undertake a PDP as part of a group than to go it alone.
- ■ You will not be unsupported – colleagues and local postgraduate dental tutors can guide you.
- ■ The standards required will be within your reach.
- ■ PDPs are liberating. Even reading this book could count as part of your development plan.

Introduction

Having read the previous chapter, you may feel a little overwhelmed! If so, don't worry, it's quite normal, but it will get easier. What you have read about represents PDPs in a highly developed form, but we all have to start somewhere and in this chapter we discuss how we can avoid drowning by dipping our toe in the water first. Therefore, we will learn how to write an abbreviated PDP and evaluate it. In reality, for all the jargon and concepts that educationists like to use, most dentists find that, having written their first development plan, they have little difficulty in coming to terms with the process and are quickly able to make their PDPs more sophisticated (and useful) in subsequent years. I am sure that this will be your experience too.

The first year

Even though you have this book and could theoretically 'fly solo', it is better to write your first plan as part of a small group. This is because you can share your anxieties with others who are at a similar stage and can help each other by talking about your needs and how they might be addressed. The group may comprise dentists from different practices or from the same practice, and there are pros and cons to both approaches. The former has the benefit of a wider range of experience and possibly of attitudes, and this can encourage colleagues to share good practice and broaden their perspectives. The latter in-house group benefits from being able to bear the needs of the practice in mind when prioritising the needs of individuals. Dentists in such groups also have a vested interest in making each other's plans successful and this can help the practice to achieve its aims. Some dentists may regard this 'pressure' as being useful while others might find it unwelcome – it rather depends on the time management and personalities of those involved.

Three meetings are proposed in the first year, the purpose of these being as follows.

- **First meeting**: to allow each dentist to identify at least one educational need and be helped to write it out in the form of a basic PDP. After this meeting, each dentist puts together the other learning needs that he has identified at this stage, and writes a plan with the guidance of his colleagues or local postgraduate dental tutors. Because this plan is the first version for the year, it is called the 'initial personal development plan'.

- **Second meeting**: dentists discuss their progress and in particular the changes (additions and deletions) that they have made to their initial development plans. Again, there is the opportunity to share concerns and ideas. In reality, at the second meeting most people are relieved to find that no one else has yet started work on their PDP! This meeting therefore provides a useful spur to activity.

   Before the final meeting, the dentists complete their development plans and reflect on the outcomes of their learning by completing an evaluation form.

- **Third meeting**: dentists discuss their evaluations and the evidence that they have collected for their portfolios and begin thinking about their learning needs for the following year's PDP.

Having a series of meetings is particularly useful in the first year when the process is new to everyone. Whether meetings continue beyond that point depends on how much colleagues gain from talking about their educational experiences, but it would be reasonable to reduce the number of meetings to two per annum. The first would be a combined evaluation of the previous year's PDP and production of an initial learning plan for the following year. The second would remain as a progress review.

Writing the initial learning plan

In the first meeting, dentists are encouraged to think about their performance. You can now try this by giving yourself ten minutes to answer the following questions. Forms for the exercises discussed are included at the end of this chapter.

- What three things do I do well?
- What three things do I do badly?

This will help you focus on what you might need to learn.

   Next, try filling in the following form as demonstrated below (a blank form is provided on page 61). This uses an example shown in the previous chapter. Give yourself 10–15 minutes for this task.

What, specifically, do I need to learn?

I need to understand a wider range of orthodontic treatments. Specifically, I want to be able to use a fixed-appliance technique.

Why do I need to learn this?

Although I use simple removable appliance orthodontics for a few patients, I don't feel confident enough to do more orthodontics.

How am I going to learn?

I could read journals and I hope to attend a course. My partner is more knowledgeable and experienced with fixed-appliance techniques and he may be willing to tutor me.

How will I use this in practice?

Instead of referring patients on, I will be able to offer a better service.

In the time available, you will probably be able to list two or three learning needs and how you would address them.

Now split into groups of two and, in turn, each talk through one learning need from your forms. The third question, *How am I going to learn?*, is usually the most important at this stage, as other people can help by suggesting resources that might be available or, better still, ones that are known to be useful. Quite often, dentists can help each other by putting colleagues in touch with a resource or even by providing personal support, especially if they have a more highly developed skill. This is the most valuable part of the meeting, and 30–45 minutes should be set aside for it. At the end of this time, you will have had a chance to think through at least one goal and answer all four questions in relation to it. As a result of this, believe it or not, you will have written your first development plan!

Some dentists prefer to continue working through their learning needs in their small groups, as described above. An alternative is to reconvene as a large group and use it to come up with ideas about how to address those learning needs that have proved problematic.

At the close of the meeting, exchange contact details with your colleagues. You are now all set to think about your other learning needs and to write these up in the form of an initial PDP.

What is expected of me?

It is important not to be too ambitious. Particularly in the first year, it is more important to get on board with the process of undertaking a simple PDP than to attempt to make it gold-plated. The object of your plan is to learn something that has the potential to be useful, so it is far better to be realistic about your goals, and thereby learn something, than to overstretch yourself and learn nothing. It is particularly pleasing if learning can be applied to practice but we recognise that this cannot always be the case. As you become familiar with the process, you will find that you are able to work backwards by selecting some improvement in dental care and then determining what skills you will need to obtain in order to bring this about.

The following pointers might help you to produce a successful first plan.

- Don't identify too many learning needs in your initial development plan. One or two are probably enough. This is because working through each goal, even the simplest, always takes longer than you anticipate. Additionally, some learning needs that demand urgent attention may arise during the course of the year and some room should be left for these in our plans.

- Try to be as specific as possible about what you need to learn, and remember that this should be a *need* and not just a *want*. If you are too general about your needs ('I need to learn more about periodontics') then you are much less likely to succeed than if your aim is more specific ('I need to learn how to interpret the values of the Debris Index').

- Say why the need is worth attending to by stating *how* it became an issue. By doing this you are in effect describing how you assessed your educational needs. If you realise where your need came from, you are also more likely to realise how your new learning will be used. For example, figures might show that you have many more failed root fillings than your partners and you might realise that this is because you feel uncomfortable about your endodontic skills. Using this to define your learning need (to learn how to fit a rubber dam) allows you to manage the condition better and reduce the number of failed procedures to the benefit of the practice and patients alike.

- When you think about how you intend to learn, try to be a little creative and avoid thinking purely about courses or lectures. Clinical dentistry is a practical skill but other interactive methods could be used, perhaps involving dental specialists in the hospital or community or even computer-aided learning. This requirement is not mandatory as different styles suit different people, but different learning methods also suit different learning needs and you may be restricting your options unnecessarily.
- Even if you are unable to say that you will be able to apply your learning directly to patient care, try to state how your PDP might make you a better practitioner.

Evaluating my first plan

At the end of the year, a simple evaluation will be required which will help to focus your mind on the value of your activities and the implications for your subsequent plan. Here is an example based on the development plan that you saw earlier. A blank form is included at the end of this chapter.

Which were the most valuable learning activities and why?

Learning from my partner. I initially felt embarrassed about admitting to my limitations, but he put me at ease. Learning in-house was much easier and less expensive than arranging time out for a course and the benefits to our own patients were immediate.

Which were the least valuable learning activities and why?

Reading the journals helped me to brush up my knowledge but did nothing to improve my confidence.

In what ways have you been able to apply your learning in practice?

I've been able to do more than just use removable appliances to tip teeth back into line.

What learning needs might you wish to carry forward to your next portfolio?

None from this area, as I feel happy (and proud!) of what I've been able to achieve.

Summary

I hope you now feel that your first PDP is within your grasp. You will find as time goes on that you will use more of the ideas and techniques you have read about in the preceding chapters, as a result of which your learning will become more focused and more effective. However, first things first. Why not have a go at writing your own PDP and discover for yourself why those who use them find them valuable.

What three things do I do well?

1

2

3

What three things do I do badly?

1

2

3

Initial PDP

What, specifically, do I need to learn?

Why do I need to learn this?

How am I going to learn?

How will I use this in practice?

Evaluation form

Which were the most valuable learning activities and why?

Which were the least valuable learning activities and why?

In what ways have you been able to apply your learning in practice?

What learning needs might you wish to carry forward to your next portfolio?

5 How to evaluate the PDP

Key points

- Once we become familiar with how to complete the plan, we will want to know how to evaluate it.
- Evaluation can look at both what we learn and how we learn.
- Evaluation can be self-directed and is helped greatly by discussion with one or more colleagues.
- The process can help us to make our learning more effective.
- We can learn how to prioritise our learning needs and use the methods that are most appropriate to them and to our learning styles.
- Ultimately, we can focus more of our time on education that leads to improvement in patient care.
- Evaluation allows us to monitor our progress towards revalidation.

Introduction

In the previous two chapters we have familiarised ourselves with the structure of the personal development plan and the PDP process. The plan has been presented as being a collection of four simple forms that between them plan, record and evaluate the part of our learning that we wish to document. Although the process is simple, it is not simplistic, as behind each element in the plan, there are educational principles that can be used to make future learning both more effective and more satisfying. This assertion is made on the basis of experience of postgraduate tutors in Sheffield, where the educational principles have been developed through peer discussion and the educational outcomes of the PDP approach have been evaluated.

In this chapter, we will look again at the elements in the plan as laid out in the PDP paperwork. For each element, the educational principles will be described. With the aid of many real examples drawn from dental practice, an interactive approach will be presented using *Checkpoints* ☑ to help us gain a deeper understanding of how these principles can be applied.

Note: this chapter can be used by learners themselves, but will be particularly valuable for those who have responsibility for helping their colleagues to improve the quality of their PDPs, such as postgraduate dental tutors.

This chapter is necessarily more involved than the introductory PDP chapters. You will get the most from it when you have gained some personal experience of writing and implementing your own PDP.

Each example that is used in the chapter provides a focus for constructive criticism but is presented in isolation of any other knowledge of the learner, his previous learning, working practices etc., all of which would have a bearing on the interpretation that might be made. To derive the maximum benefit, you should make no assumptions about the learner and offer your own observations before comparing these with the *Checkpoint discussions* made in the text.

The initial development plan

The initial plan that we have seen before in Chapter 3 is shown in Table 5.1. The highlighted areas will be discussed in turn.

Table 5.1: Initial development plan

Educational need	Reason for inclusion in development plan	Learning objectives	Activities to be used	What evidence will you keep?
What is the general area in which you need to learn?	What has motivated you to prioritise this need?	Specifically, what knowledge or ability are you hoping to gain?	What methods might you use to obtain this?	What physical evidence will you keep for your portfolio to demonstrate what you have learned?

Educational need

- **The educational need is of relevance to dental practice**

The PDP is first and foremost a *personal* development plan and although it may be influenced by external factors it should be owned and controlled by the learner. The PDP must reflect learning in the context of dental practice and, broadly speaking, this means that whatever we are proposing to learn about should have the potential of improving the care that we provide and/ or of helping us to develop professionally.

Educational needs do not have to be *directly* applicable to patient care and this is important to accept because sometimes learning results in a change of knowledge or attitude that may only later lead to a change in behaviour that can be demonstrated.

Learning within dentistry can and should be broad-based. Hence, it is just as appropriate for dentists to learn about occlusion/TMJ as it is to update themselves on injection techniques. Likewise, learning needs are not always clinical. For example, patient care may be improved as much by better communication skills as by the use of specialised dental knowledge.

- **There is a balance between the learning needs**

This means that there is a balance between:

- the learner's agenda derived from his role as a practising dentist and other posts that he might hold (for example, as a vocational trainer), as well as the wider needs of the practice
- learning that might merely inform and learning that has an immediate practical application to patient care.

The first principle reflects the fact that dentists derive their learning needs from a wide range of activities and responsibilities. PDPs may only be required to show learning for a relatively small number of hours, but they are the part of our postgraduate learning that we decide to expose to external scrutiny. It may therefore become important to be able to demonstrate, over the five-year period leading up to revalidation, that we have recognised learning needs and undertaken activity in the areas that reflect our range of responsibilities.

Note that it is not being suggested that *every* annual plan should demonstrate this balance. In practical terms, if two or three learning needs are being attended to, the scope for achieving a balance in-year is limited. However, it should be possible to think more broadly over a five-year cycle. Dentistry is primarily a practical discipline, but when we think broadly, it is important to consider other aspects of practice life – for example, communication skills, management and administration. Whatever the area of professional practice, if learning needs can be identified, they can be legitimately included in the PDP.

On the following pages, we can see examples of learning needs drawn from a wide range of activities and presented in the PDP format.

Restorative dentistry

Educational need	Reason for inclusion in development plan	Learning objectives	Activities to be used	What evidence will you keep?
Improve skills in the management of tooth surface loss.	Demographics of the practice show a relatively high number of elderly patients.	Be able to identify patients at risk.	Attend a course.	Evaluation of course.
		Know how to improve my management of tooth surface loss.	CAL program.	Assessment incorporated in the CAL program.
			Literature review.	
	Difficulties in managing older patients with significant attrition.		Develop protocols for the early and late management of tooth surface loss.	Bullet points from the dental literature.

Restorative dentistry – continued

Educational need	Reason for inclusion in development plan	Learning objectives	Activities to be used	What evidence will you keep?
Improve placement of composite restorations.	I find handling the material difficult. Patient demand for 'white fillings'.	Know how to undertake a reliable placement technique for posterior composites. Learn to use rubber dam.	Literature search. Course. Discussion with colleagues.	Audit before and after postgraduate activity. Summary of literature searches.

Prosthetics

Educational need	Reason for inclusion in development plan	Learning objectives	Activities to be used	What evidence will you keep?
I want to reduce my remakes of upper and lower dentures.	Soul-destroying to have to remake yet another denture.	Be able to identify those cases that I can do, those that I can't and need referral to a specialist.	Retrospective audit on my success/failure over past 12 months.	Audit results.
Become more confident in provision of this service.	Remove the sinking feeling when complete denture case on my day list.	Have the knowledge of a range of protocols and techniques that I can use in given circumstances.	Audit criteria might include: • counting the number of remakes in past 12 months • estimating direct loss of income and cash repaid • estimating loss of practice time.	Postgraduate course evaluation. Sample of referral letters to specialist. Case review from patient record cards. Payment schedules.
	Reduce patient discontent. Reduce lost surgery time.	Know which cases I should be referring to the local prosthodontic specialist.	Develop specialist referral guidelines with the local prosthodontist. Attend appropriate hands-on postgraduate course with the dental nurse.	

Periodontics

Educational need	Reason for inclusion in development plan	Learning objectives	Activities to be used	What evidence will you keep?
Improve periodontal monitoring.	Relatively high number of young adults in the practice population. Occasional 'surprise' periodontal problem. I'm worried about litigation if I fail to have a proper monitoring system.	Define appropriate treatment by studying guidelines.	Peer-review group discussion to consider best practice. Consult Periodontal Society guidelines. Produce practice protocol. Audit periodontal screening, looking to see that every patient seen within a 12 month period has been screened.	Audit of the clinical records. Report from peer review.

Endodontics

Educational need	Reason for inclusion in development plan	Learning objectives	Activities to be used	What evidence will you keep?
Need to improve success of root fillings within the practice.	A clinical audit revealed a depressingly high number of failed root fillings.	Know how to improve my standard of root fillings as assessed by radiographic analysis. Know how to improve the long-term survival of root-filled teeth. Be able to routinely use rubber dam in the management of posterior root fillings.	Attend hands-on course on endodontics. Attend course on the use of rubber dam. Audit radiographs of root fillings.	Evaluation of courses. Results of clinical audit.

Endodontics – continued

Educational need	Reason for inclusion in development plan	Learning objectives	Activities to be used	What evidence will you keep?
To provide more predictable success rates of endodontics using a safe technique.	A patient almost swallowed a dental file last week.	Be able to put on rubber dam successfully in 90% of cases within two minutes.	Identify someone who is good at teaching rubber dam.	Course notes.
To be able to do this under GDS regulations and still produce a good result.	I'm fed up with failed endodontic cases that result in extraction.	Know how to develop a predictable technique.	Attend a hands-on course with this person, accompanied by my nurse.	Practice protocol.
	This is embarrassing to explain to patients.	Know how to identify cases where successful endodontic treatment is unlikely.	Develop protocol to help me identify those cases I can undertake, and those I should not.	Referral guidelines produced from meeting with endodontic specialist.
	Reduces my esteem in my eyes, and those of my patients and staff.		Make contact with endodontic specialist practitioner to refer cases I don't feel able to treat and confirm referral guidelines with him.	Audit of the use of rubber dam.
	Loss of practice time and income.			
	Reduce potential litigation.		Undertake an audit on endodontic treatment in the practice.	

Minor oral surgery

Educational need	Reason for inclusion in development plan	Learning objectives	Activities to be used	What evidence will you keep?
To be able to extract teeth after failure of forceps delivery.	The specialist associate who did most of the minor oral surgery work left last month. I am now out of practice with this technique and do not feel confident. As a result, I have to refer more than I would like.	Be able to raise a surgical flap and carry out a surgical removal. Know the indications for the use of elevators.	Visit local oral surgeon and arrange one-to-one clinical training. Do some elective cases in the surgery with a suitable colleague acting as tutor/nurse. Literature review. Video training programmes.	Audit of referrals to specialists in surgical dentistry or to the oral surgery department at the dental hospital. Notes from attendance at oral surgery department. Keep a log of cases, with reflection on performance.

Local anaesthetics

Educational need	Reason for inclusion in development plan	Learning objectives	Activities to be used	What evidence will you keep?
Improve my success rate with inferior dental block.	Cause of lack of patient confidence in me when injection does not work, leading to: Potential patient dissatisfaction and loss of patient from the list. Potential medico-legal complications. Drop in my confidence and thereby further reduction in my skill in using this technique. Wasted surgery time. Loss of income.	To have an improved, reliable technique to produce at least 90% success rate at the first attempt. Identify reliable auxiliary method of local anaesthetic and be able to use this.	Audit – how bad is the problem? Peer review – share this with colleagues. Do they have solutions? Literature search to identify best practice. Postgraduate course to learn intraligamentary injection technique. Re-audit following a change of technique.	Notes from peer review. Résumé of literature search. Audit records of patients who have required dental block before and after further training.

Orthodontics

Educational need	Reason for inclusion in development plan	Learning objectives	Activities to be used	What evidence will you keep?
To provide more orthodontic treatments for patients in the practice.	I use simple removable appliance orthodontics for a few patients, but don't feel confident to do more. Patients have long waiting times to see the specialist. I also wish to develop another clinical skill, and thereby maintain my interest and enthusiasm for daily general dental practice.	To be able to undertake fixed appliance treatment in my practice.	Clinical assistantship in orthodontics at the hospital. Literature search. Join the two-year part-time GP postgraduate practical fixed appliance course.	Literature résumés. Case review. Audit of activity from the practice appointment book: are more fixed appliances being provided?

Radiography

Educational need	Reason for inclusion in development plan	Learning objectives	Activities to be used	What evidence will you keep?
Reduce the number of poor quality radiographs, especially bite-wing radiographs.	To avoid unnecessary repeat x-rays and reduce dosage to patients, self and the team.	To be able to improve quality such that 80% of radiographs are of diagnostic value.	Conduct an initial audit of performance.	Audit of records, looking for evidence of fewer retakes.
	Reduce frustration and embarrassment of retaking the radiograph, and explaining the reason to patients.	Determine the best radiograph-developing technique with the staff.	Dentist/nurse to attend a hands-on radiography course.	Evaluation of the postgraduate radiography course.
	More efficient treatment service to patients.	Be able to use film holders.	Purchase film holder and use it!	
	Improve my confidence and that of the patient.		Purchase automatic developer and make sure all staff can use it.	
	Less waste of materials and time.		Re-audit – have we improved?	

Radiography – continued

Educational need	Reason for inclusion in development plan	Learning objectives	Activities to be used	What evidence will you keep?
Need to update knowledge of radiographic regulations.	Several years since I attended a course on dental radiography and I feel out of date. I feel confused by the DoH guidance notes.	Know the up to date regulations regarding the use of dental radiographic equipment.	Attend a course on ionising radiation regulations.	Course notes.

Management and administration

Educational need	Reason for inclusion in development plan	Learning objectives	Activities to be used	What evidence will you keep?
Reduce the number of missed appointments in the practice.	Wasted surgery time, which I could use for administration or to be with my family!	Understand how best to educate patients that it is not OK to miss appointments.	Discussion with colleagues in other practices – what have they done?	Records of staff meetings.
	To reduce loss of practice income.	Decide upon the best strategy for reducing missed appointments and dealing with DNAs.	Staff meeting to discuss team approach to this problem.	Protocol of new strategy for missed appointments.
	I wish to avoid panic measures such as 'double booking'.		Communicate with patients.	Results of audit.
	Reduce stress.		Produce a practice strategy to tackle the problem and review.	
			Audit – measure how bad the problem actually is, and see how effective the strategy has been.	

Management and administration – continued

Educational need	Reason for inclusion in development plan	Learning objectives	Activities to be used	What evidence will you keep?
To motivate and support the staff	High staff turnover. I have become aware of poor morale associated with poor job prospects.	Decide upon a formal strategy to reduce staff turnover.	Discussion with partners.	Audit of staff turnover.
		Research and develop a career structure for my dental nurse.	Discussion with peer-review group.	Copy of skills training contract for dental nurse.
		Decide upon the suitability of initiatives such as Investors in People.	Take advice from the nurses' professional bodies.	
			Obtain information on suitable courses.	
			Investigate NVQ for dental nurses.	

Let us now comment on some examples of learning needs.

☑   **Checkpoint 5.1**

Based on the principles discussed on page 65, what thoughts do you have about the needs shown in Table 5.2? For this exercise, assume that these three items are the totality of the learner's PDP.

☑   **Checkpoint 5.1 discussion**

- The plan seems almost entirely dentist-centred in that there are no activities that relate directly to practice-based goals such as audit or clinical governance activities.

- With regard to improved patient care, the link with the learning needs is present but is not strong. In encouraging the learner to expand on his reasons for choosing these needs, a connection between learning and patient care might be established. For example, the learner might consider objectives that focused on clinical management, e.g. 'Improving the treatment for patients presenting with cracked tooth syndrome'. Alternatively, the learner could make sure that one of his needs specifically targeted clinical care.

- Undertaking a degree or diploma is not an uncommon activity, and is appropriate for inclusion in the PDP. However, to achieve balance, care needs to be exercised over activities that might dominate the plan. Higher learning of this sort can threaten to do so because of its very large content. A reasonable compromise, because such learning can take several years, would be to include elements from it in successive PDPs. Alternatively, it could be suggested that one educational need could consume most of the current plan with the intention that the following year's PDP would be more balanced.

- The need to keep up to date is not in question – all dentists are required to do this. However, the purpose of the initial plan is to show how dentists will meet their disclosed deficiencies. Stating that we will read the journals does not show that we have recognised a particular need, nor does it guarantee that we will learn anything! It is better to wait until we become aware through our reading that a deficiency exists, and then incorporate this need as a later addition to our plan.

Table 5.2: Initial development plan

No.	Educational need	Reason for inclusion in development plan	Learning objectives	Activities to be used	What evidence will you keep?
1	Learn about the Membership of Faculty in Dental Surgery requirements.	I wish to undertake specialist training.			
2	Develop leadership skills.	I have a role as a dental tutor that involves leading my colleagues.			
3	Keep up to date by reading the journals.	There is a need to practice evidence-based dentistry.			

- The 'need' represents a deficiency

Is the learner addressing a need or a want, i.e. is he attending to a deficiency or purely satisfying an interest? The two are not incompatible and, indeed, even if dentists have identified something that they need to learn about, they have to *want* to address this need if they are to successfully complete their plan.

As the learning plan is going to require a commitment from the learner, it is vital that he checks, as he would in practice life, that this commitment is based on a firm foundation. The foundation can be tested by asking two questions.

- Who said that I need to do this?
- What is the strength of the evidence that I need to do it?

Dentists must feel happy that they have ownership of the plan, i.e. that the priorities are their own and not purely the will of others. They must also satisfy themselves that the priorities are based on evidence of a deficiency that *they* regard as being important to correct. Some types of evidence are stronger than others. For instance, the results of a clinical audit on radiology standards might demonstrate an educational need in a way that a vague sense of unease at taking x-rays might not.

The question also gives an insight into the sources of experience from which dentists draw, which can encourage practitioners to both cultivate these further and consider why other sources are less fruitful.

The term 'deficiency' should be defined in the context of the dentist's work. Although there are core skills for all dentists, there will be areas of dental practice where a dentist needs to be more skilled than the average practitioner and some areas where a relative lack of ability is appropriate. In practice life, we would not expect to be experts in all fields and this should be reflected in our education. Of course, this argument only holds if we are able to reliably assess the skills that we *should* have in relation to our patients' needs.

Table 5.3: Initial development plan

No.	Educational need	Reason for inclusion in development plan	Learning objectives	Activities to be used	What evidence will you keep?
1	Become a vocational trainer.	The existing trainer in the practice is retiring.			
2	Learn how to remove unerupted and impacted teeth.	As this is carried out by a partner with a specialist interest, I have become rusty.			
3	To provide more predictable success rates of endodontics with a safe technique.	A patient almost swallowed a dental file last week. I'm fed up with failed endodontic cases that result in extraction.			
4	Paedodontic update.	Mums seem to prefer to bring their children to me for treatment.			

Reason for inclusion in development plan

☑ **Checkpoint 5.2**

The very act of undertaking a PDP encourages dentists to look more closely at their needs. Looking at the *reasons* for inclusion in the development plan helps to gauge both the degree of need and the motivation for learning. With this in mind, what comments do you have about the examples shown in Table 5.3?

☑ **Checkpoint 5.2 discussion**

- In the first example, the dentist needs to become a trainer, but who is this driven by? It could be that the practice requires someone to replace the outgoing trainer and the dentist has been persuaded to take on this role. Even though becoming a trainer would greatly help the dentist to develop professionally, for such a large undertaking it would be important to verify that the learner has ownership of this need.

- In the second example, the learner states that his specialist partner undertakes this work. Why then does the learner feel that *he* also needs to learn the procedure? The use of the word 'rusty' implies that he has recognised a deficiency. However, in a dental team with a range of skills, it might be more appropriate for the specialist partner rather than the learner to maintain his competence and for the learner to know when it is appropriate to refer to his colleague.

- In the third example, the dentist gives two reasons for wishing to improve his endodontics skills. The first is a good example of a significant event. Because this was a situation in which the patient could have been harmed (but fortunately was not), we could call it a 'near miss'. When patients come to harm, the motivation to put things right or to prevent a recurrence is very strong. Because significant events are powerful drivers for change, their inclusion in the plan is both appropriate and important.

  Compared with harmful events, near misses do not create the same

---

degree of distress in either ourselves or the patient and, indeed, the patient may not even be aware that a near miss has occurred. Having mopped our brow when the patient has left, the temptation is to forget the incident but this would be a mistake because today's near misses could become the harmful events of tomorrow.

Seen in this way, we should regard near misses as an opportunity, because we may not be given a second chance to avoid harm. The dentist in this example has recognised this potential and will hopefully prevent a future patient swallowing or inhaling a file. In addition, he will have converted the 'feel bad' of a near miss to the twin sense of professional pride in not having ignored the event and achievement in having improved his skills.

We should aim at some point to incorporate significant events in our development plans because they encourage us to use the powerful emotions that they generate in a positive way. Using a significant event as a 'reason for inclusion' in the plan also encourages us to be honest with ourselves about the real motivation for learning. This is illustrated by the second reason that the dentist gives for attending to this learning need. The fact that he is 'fed up' means that he has another strong reason for seeing the plan through to completion.

Compare this with other reasons that are commonly given for including an educational need, such as 'to improve patient care' or 'to improve my clinical skills'. These reasons may be sincere, but what is not clear is why the need is worthy of being *prioritised* or how motivated (and therefore committed) the dentist feels.

- In the final example, several factors emerge. The learner may be an inexperienced dentist, be responding to a significant event or have accepted responsibility for providing this service, in which case the need is appropriate. We may question whether, if he is already proficient in paedodontics, obtaining an update is really attending to the most pressing of his learning needs. Also, the fact that children are coming to this dentist *might* mean that other members of the practice are not providing an adequate service. This topic would need sensitive discussion!

- There is evidence of need

By evidence, we mean both *subjective* measures derived from reflection, questionnaires and feedback, and *objective* measures such as audit, surveys and significant event analyses. Evidence of this sort is not compulsory and, certainly in the first year, dentists may derive their needs from simple reflective exercises. However, as dentists become more experienced in planning their learning, it is likely that a short description of how educational needs have been derived will become more commonplace.

- If the dentist has a specialised role, this is being considered

Some dentists have particular responsibilities by virtue of their role as teachers, researchers or specialist dentists and, for them, there may be a need (e.g. because of appraisal or revalidation) to demonstrate that part of their continuing education is devoted to maintaining skills in these non-generalist areas.

- Addressing the need appears feasible

For the development plan to be successful it is important that it is not over-ambitious and an assessment of the feasibility of the plan can be made by looking at the workload represented by the plan and the resources required by it. The workload can be gauged by judging how ambitious the objectives seem to be and the resources can be inferred by examining the proposed activities. For example, some activities such as courses may seem like a good idea but may not be available, accessible or affordable. Also, proposing that 'every patient will receive periodontal screening within six months' may be unrealistic if manpower is not available or the patient non-attendance rate is known to be high.

Finally, we have to build in some flexibility so that we can deal with pressing educational needs as they arise. These may arise from personal experiences, such as litigation. For example, it might be claimed that because of our failure to x-ray the restored mouth of a regular patient, he has suffered unnecessary pain and the loss of a tooth. Alternatively, needs may come from external influences such as the requirement to develop a quality assurance system for clinical governance.

Learning objectives

- The learning objectives are SMART

Even for beginners, most of the process of personal development planning feels intuitive and is easily mastered. However, two elements commonly present difficulties: converting needs into useful objectives and deciding what evidence of learning should be kept.

Setting appropriate learning objectives is not an academic exercise designed to frustrate the learner, but as we will see is fundamental to success in the PDP spiral. Objectives define the desired outcomes of the learning process; there may be only one if the educational need is small or there may be several if the need is larger and has to be broken down into a number of manageable steps.

These objectives can be thought of as the staging posts in meeting the aim, and good objectives are said to be **SMART**, meaning that they are:

- Specific: clear and concise.
- Measurable: written as verbs (e.g. know, apply, plan, etc.) rather than as 'woolly' objectives (e.g. feel more confident, become aware of, appreciate, etc.) which cannot be easily defined or measured.
- Achievable: by ensuring that resources (e.g. expertise, time and funding) are available and that the goals are attainable.
- Relevant to the aim.
- Time-bound: with the date for completion being both explicit and realistic.

In practice, objectives often state the new ability that the learner is seeking to acquire. This may be in the following forms.

- New *knowledge* that the learner requires in order to meet his overall educational need – for example, 'to know the criteria and standards for the Investors in People award'.
- Sometimes, the objective may refer to a practical *skill* – e.g., 'to be able to fit an implant'.
- Alternatively it can be an *attitude*, such as 'to understand the value of

allowing shared decision-making in the dental team'. Whatever the objective, being specific about it is the most important feature.

Aims and objectives sometimes get confused with each other, but an aim is the ultimate purpose of our activity and the objectives are those tasks which need to be completed in order to achieve that aim. Suppose that our aim was to take a holiday in Peru. Our objectives would then include specific tasks such as buying the airline tickets, obtaining foreign currency and having our holiday vaccinations.

With the PDP, our aim is usually written as an educational need and may be large and relatively unfocused. Writing clear objectives allows us to plan how we will meet our aim. In this way, we can convert a nebulous goal into a series of manageable steps that between them will ensure that we succeed in achieving what we set out to do. Very often, when plans fail they do so because the objectives have been poorly thought out and as a result become difficult to achieve or irrelevant to the original aim. To illustrate this, look at Table 5.4.

Table 5.4: Personal development plan

Educational need	Learning objectives
To have better radiographic procedures.	1 Have a look at the recent literature. 2 Beer review! 3 Produce a protocol.

If we were to carry through these learning objectives, could we be sure of meeting our aim? To help decide upon our objectives, it is useful to ask:

- 'What do I want to be able to do that I can't do now?' and
- 'How will I know when I've got there?'

One way of thinking about how to *phrase* our objectives is to complete the sentence: 'At the end of this process I will . . .'

In doing so, the second half of the sentence will often contain a verb like 'write' (for example, a guideline), 'know', 'summarise' and so on. This phrase will usually provide a form of words that we can use in our plan.

Now look at Table 5.5, in which the need is the same but the objectives have been modified.

Table 5.5: Personal development plan

Educational need	Learning objectives
To have better radiographic procedures.	1 Decide upon an appropriate system for quality control. 2 Have a core of knowledge certificate. 3 Know how to audit continuing care.

Try comparing these objectives with those offered in Table 5.4. If you were to implement the revised objectives, you would be better placed to meet your need than in the original example and this is because the objectives are SMART. Can you identify in what ways?

When we write the educational priorities for our PDPs, it is usually intended that we complete the objectives within the following 12 months, which includes the time needed to fill in the forms and evaluate our learning. Because the plan is limited to a year, each of the objectives could be said to be time-bound. Some dentists prefer to commit themselves to shorter deadlines within the year and, if this is done, we need to be realistic about the timescale for each aim that we define. Giving ourselves too little time runs the risk of leaving us exhausted and demotivated; giving ourselves too much may deprive us of any sense of urgency and the task may never be completed.

Whether we set intermediate goals or not, we need to remember that although we will be working towards several educational objectives simultaneously, we may need to complete some ahead of others. For example, if there has been a significant event we may consider it to be more important to learn how to use a rubber dam than to improve our skills with managing tooth surface loss.

☑ **Checkpoint 5.3**

What comments would you make about the objectives in Table 5.6?

Table 5.6: Initial development plan

No.	Educational need	Reason for inclusion in development plan	Learning objectives	Activities to be used	What evidence will you keep?
1	Improve my minor oral surgery skills.	I'm concerned that my patients may not be adequately managed.	Feel more confident about my clinical ability.		
2	Investigate how feasible it is to become a paperless practice.	• Many practices are doing this, and our paper records are becoming unwieldy. • Patients are commenting that we seem to be behind the times.	Talk with a colleague who has made the change.		
3	To improve the standards of my root canal work.	As a new dentist, I feel that I lack experience in this area.	Undertake a case review of the next few patients that I treat.		

☑ **Checkpoint 5.3 discussion**

- The first learning objective seems rather vague. Feeling more confident is an outcome that would apply to most learning needs, but it is not a specific objective. It does not indicate what *ability*, rather than feeling, the learner is seeking to achieve and gives no indication of how he would know when he had achieved his objective. In reality, how would the dentist know when he was 'confident enough' and how valid is this as an end-point of learning? Unfortunately, competence decays far more quickly than confidence!

    If SMART objectives are not set, there is the risk that the learner will take far longer to reach the destination, or worse still go off track and miss it entirely, leaving him with feelings of disappointment and frustration.

    It is important to be honest, and admitting to large areas of 'weakness' is a valuable first step that should be encouraged. This could serve as a starting point and the process of setting specific objectives could then be used to help refine the area that needs prioritising. Thus for the first example it might transpire that learning how to extract teeth after the failure of forceps delivery and when to use elevators are the main areas of minor oral surgery that are of interest, and each of these could then be written as SMART objectives.

- In the second example, the objective 'talk with a colleague' is not SMART and is really an activity or learning method rather than an objective. The idea of talking to someone who has had experience of the proposed change is perfectly sensible, but it would help learning to be more effective and time-efficient if the learner could decide in advance what his main concerns were in relation to becoming paperless. On the basis of this, the dentist could then decide what issues he wished to raise with his colleague. For example, he might want to talk about the resources required to become paperless, the logistics of change, legal aspects, confidentiality, how records are made available for referrals, etc. Each of these would make a suitable objective and the discussion, when it occurred, would have more chance of being productive.

- In the last example, 'undertake a case review' is again an activity rather than a learning objective. If this was our development plan, we might think about what we were hoping to gain from this activity and this could suggest certain standards in endodontics that we might wish to measure ourselves against. Conversely, the process of reflection might indicate that we were not sure what those standards (for example, diagnosis, access, debridement and shaping) should be. In either event, we would have the basis for establishing some clearer objectives by which we could meet our overall aim of improving our management of patients who required root canal treatment.

Activities to be used

Having produced SMART objectives, we next need to ask ourselves how these will be achieved. Our answer will, in effect, outline our learning activities.

At the time that the initial learning plan is written, the exact activities to be used may not be clear and will almost certainly change as learning proceeds. It is important that the initial learning plan indicates that the learner has some idea about how he would *start* to learn, the priority being that his chosen activities seem appropriate to the stated objectives. As learning proceeds, the activities may change, influenced by the availability of resources such as appropriate tutors, courses, the recommendations of colleagues and our preferred learning styles.

Activities are otherwise known as learning methods, and as a secondary issue we might look at the range of methods being used. Some learners prefer to work in isolation or learn passively by going to lectures. However, as postgraduate education becomes increasingly multidisciplinary, we might wish to think about using interactive activities such as talking to colleagues, working in groups or using team-based approaches.

There is no right or wrong way to learn and the important point is to choose a method of learning that suits the purpose defined by our objectives. For transferring information and getting a quick 'update', we may prefer solitary methods of learning, e.g. didactic teaching such as reading a book or attending a postgraduate lecture. On the other hand, for putting information into the context of our practice, as with learning how to alter our case management in the light of new guidelines, it may be better to choose an interactive method such as peer discussion. Much of our education is enhanced if it is interactive and learning with our colleagues allows us to gain insights that may not have occurred to us, as well as helping us to apply our learning more effectively. Our chosen companions for learning may be other dentists, but the dental team is wider than the dentists alone. Nowadays, increasing importance is attached to multidisciplinary learning, i.e. learning facilitated by and shared between members of the team.

The learning method also needs to be appropriate to the attribute we hope to gain. Hence knowledge can be acquired from a book but if we were trying to gain a skill such as using a variable taper crown-down technique, we would do better to gain practical experience with a tutor or work on extracted teeth.

Some examples of methods that we could use are shown in Box 5.1.

Box 5.1 Learning methods

Reading	for ourselves or as part of a journal club using books, journals and literature searches
Lectures	the better ones having clear objectives with an opportunity for discussion
Meetings and discussions	with partners, colleagues (e.g. peers, consultants, postgraduate advisers, tutors, mentors, etc.), members of the healthcare team and the wider public
Workshops	small-group, task-orientated work
Courses	including hands-on, distance learning by post or electronically via the Internet
Personal tuition	perhaps being taught a practical skill by a colleague
Work experience	e.g. clinical assistantships
Audit	either conducted by ourselves or by learning lessons from audit conducted by others
Research	usually with support, often as part of a research group
Computer-assisted learning	e.g. Internet searching using search engines such as Medline, being part of an email discussion group, using interactive packages on the Internet or CD-ROM CAL packages

In choosing the methods, we will have in mind our previous experiences and may tend to favour those approaches that worked for us in the past. This might be because we enjoyed that way of learning, because it was feasible or simply because it achieved results.

Learning methods that have proved their effectiveness by leading to change deserve to be prioritised in this way. However, we will not know all the possible methods and the pros and cons of each approach, and for this reason it can be helpful to supplement our experience with the advice of colleagues when deciding which educational methods would be most appropriate. Between them, colleagues will have a wider range of learning styles and therefore of favoured methods, and will know which courses, speakers, etc., are worth using and which should be avoided. In addition to providing advice, colleagues can turn out to be good tutors, and it is remarkable how even a small group of dentists can significantly further each other's education.

☑ **Checkpoint 5.4**

Look at the activities in the learning plan shown in Table 5.7. To what degree do they reflect the principles discussed?

☑ **Checkpoint 5.4 discussion**

- The first two activities lack a clear potential for interactive learning and this is an issue that could be raised. It might be that the learner prefers to work alone, but it may be that he or she feels insecure or isolated.

  A more appropriate way to learn might be to go to a hands-on course with the dental nurse. Rather than learn from a secondary care specialist, it would be even better for the course provider to be someone from general dental practice, e.g. a specialist dental practitioner. Such a person would have the appropriate skills and would understand the particular difficulties that a generalist might face and how these could be overcome.

- The second activity seems rather passive for the acquisition of such a practical skill. Using a book is unlikely to be as effective as being shown how to give the injection. It would help to explore why the learner had chosen this activity rather than other methods, such as learning from a colleague or attending a clinical skills course. It might be that he feels inadequate or fears being embarrassed, both of which are important issues to explore sensitively before commenting on the choice of activity or suggesting suitable alternatives.

- Some of the same comments apply to the third activity. The learner has expressed his feelings of inadequacy compared to his colleagues, and may feel that they would not be suitable teachers. This could be discussed and hopefully overcome, as colleagues are often happy to help each other if invited to do so. In general, many distance-learning courses are of high-quality, especially in this computer age where interactive methods are used, and such a course might be appropriate for this learner. The learner stated that his need was in relation to the use of the practice computer, and we might check that the content of the course was addressing this need.

What evidence will you keep?

Being asked for 'proof' can seem threatening and there is a need to achieve a balance between keeping an educational focus for the PDP and using it as a means to demonstrate accountability to such people as appraisers and the GDC. Here are some guidelines that can help.

- **There is evidence of learning and sometimes evidence of application**

Evidence comes in different grades and, in the most basic form, it may be little more than proof that the learner has engaged in the learning process. For example, if time is being claimed for non-verifiable CPD, we may need to produce evidence such as a record of the hours spent in completing our objectives. The activity summary of the PDP can serve this purpose.

An improvement on this would be to produce evidence arising from reflection on educational activities as described below. In its most advanced form, evidence refers to the application of learning, as might be demonstrated through a change in practice. This goal is certainly important, but may not always be within the power of the learner to deliver, perhaps because it requires the efforts of others to achieve, requires additional resources or

Table 5.7: Initial development plan

No.	Educational need	Reason for inclusion in development plan	Learning objectives	Activities to be used	What evidence will you keep?
1	Update myself with the new nickel-titanium endodontic system.	These new systems appear to have revolutionised the practice of endodontics and it appears that this is the way forward.	To know how to use this system, especially for molar endodontics.	Go to an evening lecture at the dental hospital.	
2	Improve my success rate with local anaesthesia.	Patients lose confidence in me when the inferior dental block doesn't work.	Know how to use the intraligamentary injection technique as an auxiliary method.	Look at some photographs on injection technique.	
3	Learn how to use the practice computer.	The computer in my consulting room has been updated. My dental colleagues seem to be experts, but I feel ignorant about using a PC.	• To be able to use the Internet, particularly for email. • To be able to use the word processor.	Enrol in a distance-learning course that teaches computer skills.	

cannot easily be measured. To illustrate these points, we know that improving oral health needs co-operative patients as well as good dentistry. Also, learning about the needs of the elderly may make us more understanding as dentists but might prove difficult to demonstrate.

- **Evidence arises from mainstream activity**

The most useful evidence is that which helps us to get the most from our educational activity as well as serving the needs of accountability. This means that, wherever possible, evidence should arise from our mainstream activity rather than be produced solely for assessors.

For example, if our learning need was 'to improve the aftercare of patients who are provided with dentures', we may decide to produce a patient information leaflet covering how to clean the dentures and what to do in the event of a fracture. This would be invaluable to the practice as well as providing good evidence of learning. Other examples of such evidence include audit work or the production of administrative protocols. For those dentists that spend time presenting ideas or educating others, the material that is produced for this purpose, such as handouts, overhead projector slides or meeting notes, could be used as evidence.

- **Proof of reflection**

Sometimes evidence does not arise quite so directly from learning, and in these circumstances we can produce evidence that presents our thoughts about what we have learned. This is sometimes called 'proof of reflection' as distinct from 'proof of action'. We often learn through reading, and it is in no one's interest to keep the primary material that we have read – we would soon run out of filing cabinets in any case! Instead, we could do any of the following:

- highlight the important points in the text
- write down the reference and produce bullet points of the material thought relevant
- write a few lines on how the new information might influence our future practice.

Because of the high baseline level of knowledge, practising dentists rarely gain more than a few key points from each article. Hence considerable time spent reading may be summarised in only a few sentences and this may surprise or even disappoint learners, who might be expecting to keep reams of material. The resulting portfolio of evidence may not look so impressive in terms of sheer bulk, but dentists should be reassured that quality not quantity is the key.

Where learning has occurred through attending a lecture or course, going to a meeting, etc., evidence of reflection might be an evaluation in terms of what was learned or how our practice might be influenced by the event. This could be written as a learning log. Table 5.8 is an example of such a log that shows how proof of reflective learning could be provided from a range of activities.

Many educational meetings that we attend are advertised without clear objectives. This is unfortunate because having objectives of learning can both focus the efforts of the presenter and allow dentists to decide beforehand whether the objectives are relevant to their learning needs and therefore whether the meeting is worth attending. The evaluation form on pages 100–1 shows how tutors and learners can benefit from having clear objectives that can be evaluated. This form is far more useful educationally than the certificates of attendance that we usually collect at dental meetings. A blank form, which you might consider using for your own meetings, is provided at the end of this chapter.

Table 5.8: Learning log

Date	Activity	Subject area	Learning aim	What did I learn?	How could I apply what I have learned in practice?
2/10/02	Peer-review meeting	Aesthetic restoration	To learn to use the newer dental materials properly	Failure of my composite restorations sometimes occurs because dental curing lights are not always effective for these materials if the light intensity drops	1 Check my lights with a meter more regularly 2 Change the curing light bulbs more often
12/11/02	GDP clinical assistant session in local hospital	Complete dentures	To understand reasons for failure of retention of complete upper dentures	Most complete upper dentures made in general dental practice are inadequately extended in the post-dam region	Check post-dam extension of patient's existing dentures *before* making a replacement.
12/12/02	Hands-on section 63 meeting	Endodontics	To improve quality of root canal preparations	Apical obturation cannot be successfully carried out unless preceded by coronal preparation	To use wider files in the coronal portion before proceeding to the use of my usual smaller ones in the apical region (crown-down rather than step-back)

Evaluation form for a workshop on the PDP

Thanks for attending the workshop. You can keep the upper part of this form for your portfolio.

Compared to what I previously knew, what have I learned?

I didn't have much idea previously. Although I tried to write a PDP before, I wasn't sure how to complete it, so it remained in a drawer!
I now know how to write a simple plan and implement it.

How might this change my practice?
(How might it change the way I think or behave?)

I might have a go at writing a PDP, but if I do, I will want to do it along with my two partners. Potentially, the PDP might make me think about educating myself for the future rather than just reacting to my current 'failings'.

If it would not, what are the reasons?
(e.g. is there not enough evidence to change, is it not a priority or are there resources that I require?)

I will need time and the support of my colleagues to make this happen. If I could claim the time spent on the PDP toward my verifiable hours, that would be a help.

. . . Please complete the lower part and hand in to course presenter . . .

This workshop had the following objectives.

1 Understand the PDP paperwork for dentists.
2 Understand the PDP spiral.
3 Identify two personal development needs.
4 Write one personal development need in the initial development plan format.
5 Decide how PDPs will be used in vocational training.

Using the scales below, score the extent to which these objectives were achieved:

1	Not at all	1	2	3	4	⑤	Fully achieved
2	Not at all	1	2	3	4	⑤	Fully achieved
3	Not at all	1	2	3	④	5	Fully achieved
4	Not at all	1	2	3	4	⑤	Fully achieved
5	Not at all	1	2	③	4	5	Fully achieved

In what way could this meeting have been improved?

Very useful. More time to discuss the implications for VT would have been useful, but otherwise no complaints!

As a means of raising our awareness, reflection is very powerful and formalising it in this way can help us to capture the lessons learned in a way that 'just thinking about it' cannot.

- **Certificates of learning**

Although they are the traditional method of proving CPD, certificates of attendance are not adequate in themselves, as they are merely proof of attendance not proof of learning. It would be better to complete a proforma such as an entry on the learning log or an evaluation form as shown earlier in this chapter.

Occasionally, certificates are issued that do provide confirmation that learning has taken place. Examples include certification that a dentist has been trained in a particular skill (e.g. sedation), certificates of satisfactory completion of distance-learning courses, and diplomas and degrees awarded by educational bodies. All of these are valid forms of evidence, but if dentists are engaged in certified forms of learning, they should not feel obliged to obtain the relevant end-point certificate in order to demonstrate learning. They may choose to set themselves intermediate goals and produce evidence of what they have learned.

For example, as discussed below, a dentist studying to be a specialist orthodontist could set a more achievable goal of being able to place fixed appliances in some of the simpler IOTN (index of treatment needs) cases. For this, he could use his anonymised case records as evidence.

☑   **Checkpoint 5.5**

Consider the evidence column in Table 5.9. How appropriate do you feel it is in relation to the learning needs shown and what suggestions would you make to the learner?

☑   **Checkpoint 5.5 discussion**

- For the first need, a series of certificates is merely proof of attendance. Better evidence could relate back to the learning objectives and might include pre- and post-operative records of treatment undertaken with fixed appliances, e.g. study models and clinical photographs.
- In the second need, photocopies are not as useful as highlighted text or bullet points. One method is to cite the reference and then make a note of the key points.
- The third need, however laudable, is very ambitious and rather than set such a high target of achieving the diploma, the learner could think of another that lies en route to the ultimate goal. For example, the learner could decide to improve his clinical photographic skills, in which case the evidence could be the photographs that he submits in his case reports.

Amending the development plan

We have previously seen how the PDP provides an opportunity to be proactive with our learning. However, because the plan is written at the start of the year, we cannot be certain that the priorities defined in the initial development plan will maintain their importance as time progresses. Our priorities may change, perhaps prompted by practice or locality demands or by significant events relating to clinical care. In addition, our original learning

Table 5.9: Initial development plan

No.	Educational need	Reason for inclusion in development plan	Learning objectives	Activities to be used	What evidence will you keep?
1	Develop further expertise in orthodontics.	Personal interest and because at present we cannot provide this service within the practice.	Be able to place fixed appliances in some of the simpler IOTN cases.	Attend hands-on courses.	Certificates of attendance.
2	Update on endodontic techniques.	Failed molar endodontics.	To carry out fewer extractions of root-treated teeth on my patients.	Read a recent series of articles on endodontics from the BDJ.	Photocopies of the articles that I have read.
3	To pass the Membership of Faculty of General Dental Practitioners.	The qualification would help me to become a postgraduate tutor/vocational training adviser.	Know the factual material required. Be able to demonstrate clinical photographic skills.	Read the dental journals. Revise from the textbooks. Attend a course.	MFGDP diploma.

needs may have to be deferred because the resources required to meet them (lectures, courses, etc.) are not available. Therefore, we may wish to change our plan, and such amendments (additions and deletions) are not only 'allowed' but are inevitable and demonstrate the responsiveness of our learning to the context of our working lives.

Being aware of the need to allow for flexibility in the plan means that we should not commit ourselves to a large number of learning needs at the start of the year. For example, some dentists like to learn reactively (rather than prospectively) from needs that are identified in the course of daily practice. They therefore leave sufficient time in their annual plan, e.g. a quarter of their accredited hours, to make use of these opportunities as they arise.

We will have put a lot of thought into writing our initial plan, and if we are to make wholesale changes it will be important to make sure that the integrity of the plan is not compromised. We could do this by asking the following questions about the amendments.

1 Are educational needs that we initially considered important (e.g. on the basis of poor care or even patient harm) being abandoned?
2 Is there an obstacle to learning, such as a resource or training issue, that could be addressed?
3 Is the balance of the plan, as discussed earlier, being compromised? If so, does this matter?
4 Is the amended plan feasible in the given timescale?
5 Will the plan still meet the needs of revalidation?

Therefore, although amendments can be freely made, we should be prepared to justify them if required. To make this easier, the PDP paperwork that we have studied contains a page for amendments such as the example shown in Table 5.10.

☑ **Checkpoint 5.6**

We have previously looked at how to comment on additions to the learning plan and therefore we will now take the opportunity to look at examples in Table 5.10 of *deletions* from the plan. Examining these, what thoughts do you have about them and what might you suggest to the learner?

Table 5.10: Personal development plan: amendments

Educational need	Reason for including/ removing from development plan	Development objectives for additions	Activities to be used for additions	What evidence will you keep?
To produce an effective cross-infection control policy.	I removed this need in order to learn how to bleach teeth.			
To be able to use the word processor.	This was removed because the book that came with the PC was not very helpful.			

☑ **Checkpoint 5.6 discussion**

- For the first deletion, the concern is that the original educational need seemed significant in terms of patient care or, in this case, the potential to cause patient harm. Although learning how to bleach teeth might be important, we might wish to check that the original need was not being overlooked, which it might be because, for example, the dentist was concerned about the cost implications of buying an autoclave or losing treatment time and therefore income.

- With the second deletion, it is clear that the dentist found that his learning method was inadequate for the task. Perhaps another approach such as learning from a colleague or attending a workshop might be better. Alternatively, the learner may feel insecure about using the computer and would prefer to back-pedal on his commitment. The desire to improve IT skills is a very common learning need and being taught by someone who is not an expert but a recent novice can help to build confidence.

- Sometimes, as possibly in the second example, the learner may decide that the learning need still requires attention but needs to be approached in a different way. In that case, tackling the subject could be deferred perhaps to the next PDP.

Evaluating the learning process

Once the plan is complete, it is considered important to evaluate both the outcomes of learning and the process of learning itself, the purpose being to help to make our future learning more effective. The technique is one of self-evaluation, using questions such as the following. An example of a completed form using these questions is given on pages 110–11.

How did we identify our learning needs for this PDP, and what other methods might we include in our next PDP?

Many dentists determine their needs intuitively and therefore may not recognise that assessing learning needs is a skill that can be learned. A range of techniques, both subjective (e.g. reflection, feedback and questionnaires) and objective (e.g. clinical audit) can be used. They have the potential to give us insights on our performance in different areas of practice or to look at our performance in one area from different perspectives. For example, the standard of our consultations could be gauged both by auditing our punctuality in keeping to appointment times and by using a patient satisfaction questionnaire. Thinking about ways in which we identify our needs helps us to identify the techniques that we use, and can help to broaden the range of techniques that we employ in the future.

Which objectives were easiest/most difficult to achieve and why?

The importance of writing SMART objectives has been stressed, but it is not intuitive and therefore can be difficult to learn. Reflecting upon those objectives that either worked, or did not work well, is a good way of demonstrating to ourselves the link between successful outcomes of learning and the use of SMART objectives.

If our objectives were not achieved, we could speculate on the reasons for this and on how we might achieve success in the future. It might have been that the objectives we set were unrealistic, resources were not available or commitment was lacking.

Which were the most/least valuable learning activities and why?

As experienced learners, we have our own favourite learning methods that reflect our educational needs as well as our personalities. Although educationalists sometimes assume that certain methods (e.g. talk and chalk lectures) are bad and others (e.g. small-group work) are good, this is debatable and the important factor is not the method itself but whether it is effective in helping us to achieve our objectives.

Colleagues may suggest other routes to learning. For instance, because the perspectives and feedback of others can be so illuminating, interactive methods could be suggested to dentists who seem to learn mainly in isolation.

Broadening the range of methods employed can be useful, but it may be equally appropriate to continue with a learning method (e.g. computer-assisted learning) that we have found works for us.

In what ways have we been able to apply our learning to practice?

The ultimate aim of the PDP process is to learn *and* to be able to apply that learning to practice, preferably in a way that produces benefits for patients.

If improvements occurred, it is helpful to put them into context by showing how they are an advance on previous practice. If learning was not applied, it is just as important to discuss why this was either not appropriate or not possible.

This element of evaluation is likely to be particularly important to outsiders (including members of the lay public) who may be authorised to look at our plans. The laity may be less concerned with what the dentist has experienced through education than in what the patients have gained.

Are there any learning needs that we wish to carry forward to the next PDP?

On reflection, we may wish to carry some existing needs forward, perhaps with new objectives, or to address new areas of need uncovered while undertaking the PDP. Each PDP should inform future plans by helping to make the process of learning more effective, but should not automatically dictate the content of these plans. Therefore, we should not feel obliged to take educational needs forward from one year's plan to the next.

Self-evaluation is conducted by answering the questions discussed above, perhaps using a proforma such as that shown at the end of Chapter 3. To gain the maximum value these evaluations can be usefully discussed in a group, as there may be lessons that have a wider application. For instance, a positive outcome of learning due to the use of a good resource deserves to be more widely known. On the other hand, if barriers are identified such as a lack of support or funding, these could be addressed and overcome, especially if the group discussing their PDPs are members of the same practice.

Evaluation can serve as a springboard to future learning, and it may be that in time to come such a meeting could encompass both evaluation of the

Table 5.11: Development plan: initial version

Educational need	Reason for inclusion in development plan	Learning objectives	Activities to be used	What evidence will you keep?
Antibiotic prophylaxis.	I don't feel confident about the conditions for which I should be recommending prophylaxis against infective endocarditis.	1 Know which conditions are important. 2 Know which antibiotic regimes to recommend. 3 Know how to alert the dentist of the need for prophylaxis.	1 Reading. 2 Talk with partners and manager about disease register/record keeping/use of computer prompts.	Audit patients with predisposing conditions for infective endocarditis: have they received appropriate treatment?

previous year's PDP and consideration of next year's initial learning plan. For many health professionals, the appraisal interview provides such an opportunity in a one-on-one discussion with a peer.

☑ **Checkpoint 5.7**

Bearing this discussion in mind, look at the initial development plan in Table 5.11 and the associated evaluation in Box 5.2, which were used in Chapter 3. What comments would you make about the learner's evaluation that might help with his future learning?

Box 5.2 Development plan: evaluation

How did you identify your learning needs for this PDP, and what other methods might you include in your next PDP?

Mostly by self-reflection. I did an audit to confirm that I was using antibiotics appropriately, and the audit technique is one that I could use next year to determine where my needs lie.

Which objectives were easiest to achieve and why?

Learning about the indications for antibiotics – just a matter of looking it up in a book.

Which objectives were most difficult to achieve and why?

Sorting out how I could make use of the computer to prompt me in surgery, because lots of other people were involved and I didn't feel confident about using the computer.

Which were the most valuable learning activities and why?

Talking with the practice manager about how to use the practice computer. She was patient with me and I felt a sense of achievement at being able to do more than just switch it on.

Which were the least valuable learning activities and why?

Discussing the protocol with the partners. Not everyone was enthusiastic and they were concerned that setting up the disease register was expensive and unnecessary.

In what ways have you been able to apply your learning to practice?

I've been alerted when antibiotic was needed at a time in advance of the consultation when appropriate advice could be given.

What benefits to your patients do you feel have occurred as a result of your learning?

Wasted consultations have been avoided and patients have been properly protected when they have attended for treatment such as scale and polish.

   They have also commented favourably on our computerised system which they say makes the practice seem more 'up to date'.

Are there any learning needs that you wish to carry forward to your next PDP?

Implementing my plan make me recognise my ignorance at using the computer and I need to prioritise this next year.

☑ Checkpoint 5.7 discussion

- The learner has used an important technique to identify his needs. The value of reflection is widely appreciated, but time for this activity is seldom put by and having a PDP encourages dentists to routinely reflect upon their work. The learner happened to use an objective method (audit) to show how his practice had changed. As he points out, audit can also be used prospectively to identify a problem area of which he might not have been aware.
- SMART objectives are the cornerstone of achieving success in the PDP. We could have predicted that the first two objectives in the development plan would have been easy to meet because they are both

SMART and this turned out to be the learner's experience. The third objective proved more difficult because it was less Achievable. The dentist found that the involvement of many people and his own lack of confidence with the computer were barriers to achieving his objective. This may not have been predictable, but in future he might modify his approach perhaps by allowing more time for objectives that require teamwork. His honesty in admitting to insecurity with the use of the computer is useful because in doing so he has identified an important learning need.

- The dentist valued the assistance of the practice manager. He will have experienced the usefulness of one-on-one learning but, in addition, his attitude toward learning from other team members may have been improved.

- The discussion with the partners appears to have been an unhappy one. We can understand the perspectives of both sides – the partner who has put a lot of work into a new protocol and the colleagues who do not feel motivated to the same degree. The learner's comments remind us that because dentists work in teams, changes to the way the practice operates may not happen unless people feel committed to them. As the rest of the evaluation shows, the dentist's colleagues did not stand in the way of progress but the learner might like to think about how the sense of ownership could be increased next time around. One method is to have a planning meeting at the start of the year and then jointly decide the aims and apportion the work that needs to be done. This ensures that colleagues feel jointly committed and supportive of the work undertaken by individuals.

- Despite the difficulties, the learner has achieved his aim and is being appropriately forewarned of the need for prophylaxis.

- Learning does not always produce direct improvements in patient care, but it has done so in this instance. The benefits have been wider than the learner might have anticipated, as his comments about patient feedback indicate. This experience may encourage the learner to see patient feedback in a positive light and to plan to make use of it in the future.

- New learning needs are often uncovered during the course of completing the plan, but this does not mean that they necessarily have to be attended to. It would have been quite appropriate for the learner to say this, but in this example, he feels that the need to improve his IT skills is a personal priority and is worthy of being carried forward.

Summary

Evaluation of the PDP may seem threatening, but it has the capacity to help make our learning more effective. Currently, we do not think concretely about the value of the hours we spend in CPD and whether these hours do any good. Looking at the plan and its outcomes helps us to choose those areas that are genuine rather than imagined priorities and to think more carefully about the ultimate beneficiaries of our efforts. If our learning is intended to benefit our patients as well as ourselves, has it done so? If not, perhaps we should modify our approach next time around.

As we have seen in this chapter, learning to modify our plans as a result of self-evaluation is the cornerstone to making progress in the PDP spiral and to producing the appropriate evidence of learning that will be expected of us.

Evaluation form

Thanks for attending the meeting. You can keep the upper part of this form for your portfolio.

Compared to what I previously knew, what have I learned?

How might this change my practice?
(How might it change the way I think or behave?)

If it would not, what are the reasons?
(e.g. is there not enough evidence to change, is it not a priority or are there resources that I require?)

. . . Please complete the lower part and hand in to course presenter . . .

This workshop had the following objectives.

1

2

3

4

Using the scales below, score the extent to which these objectives were achieved:

1 Not at all	1	2	3	4	5	Fully achieved
2 Not at all	1	2	3	4	5	Fully achieved
3 Not at all	1	2	3	4	5	Fully achieved
4 Not at all	1	2	3	4	5	Fully achieved

In what way could this meeting have been improved?

6 PUNs & DENs

What are PUNs & DENs?

How can individuals use them?

How do we use PUNs & DENs in our consultations?

How could the practice team use PUNs & DENs?

Summary

Key points

- The PUNs & DENs approach is self-directed, and is usually based on the consultation.
- It is derived directly from what we do.
- Although it quickly highlights deficiencies, we should also remember our strengths.
- Not all PUNs lead to DENs
- PUNs can be established more widely, for example through audit.
- Involving others makes the process less subjective, increases its value and makes it more fun!
- Collating the PUNs of individuals allows the Team Educational Needs to be established.

What are PUNs & DENs?

Dr Richard Eve first described PUNs & DENs as a mechanism by which professionals can identify their educational needs by analysing their activity in clinical practice. His idea was that many of our clinical encounters result in a patient's needs not being met. Some of these *Patients' Unmet Needs* (PUNs) may be due to the dentist's lack of knowledge or skill, and identifying them allows us to define the *Dentist's Educational Needs* (DENs).

We've all had the experience in surgery – sometimes several times a day – of thinking 'I must go and find out about that'. On occasions, we are aware that if we *had* a particular ability we would not need to refer the patient for an opinion or for a procedure. With the PUNs & DENs approach, we learn to *record* these experiences and use them to identify and prioritise what we need to learn.

The technique has some strengths and weaknesses.

Strengths

Being based on the bedrock of dental practice, the clinical encounter, greatly increases the validity of the technique as the areas of educational need that it identifies are derived first-hand from what we do with our patients. It is simple to use, immediate and relatively unobtrusive and makes us aware of problem areas that we might otherwise simply ignore.

The use of this method doesn't cause us much anxiety as it is usually a form of self-evaluation. Additionally, the act of thinking about and recording PUNs makes us more patient-centred and this in itself may improve our consulting skills. Recording PUNs also makes it more likely that we will act on them.

Compared with other forms of evaluation, many DENs can be quickly addressed, for example by looking something up in a book or asking a colleague for advice, and therefore this approach can rapidly produce benefit for our patients and for ourselves.

Weaknesses

It is *subjective* and is dependent on our skill at assessing and disclosing a patient's need, our ability to recognise a need once disclosed and our honesty in admitting that the need was unmet. Because each consultation may disclose PUNs & DENs, many educational needs may quickly be uncovered and this may prove demotivating if we find it difficult to sort the wheat from the chaff. The record made is a negative one, in that it is an account of all the things that we did *not* do and what this might indicate about our deficiencies. To compensate for this we need to learn to *recognise our strengths* at the same time as recording our PUNs & DENs.

The process of recording PUNs & DENs needs to take place either after each consultation (be it for examination or treatment) or at the end of surgery while the events are still fresh in our minds. This will therefore make our surgeries last a little longer. In practice, we use several techniques to identify our educational needs and therefore it is inappropriate (and impossible!) to record PUNs & DENs after each surgery. We can gain most by planning to use it on occasions, giving ourselves sufficient time. We can thereby learn the technique and repeat the process occasionally rather than routinely. Many people find that once they are used to using the approach, they automatically become aware of important needs as they arise, rather than ignore them as they might have done before. They then begin to think in terms of whether and how the needs could be met.

How can individuals use them?

Using PUNs & DENs is a simple approach with obvious charm, but care needs to be taken that it does not become simplistic. There is the danger that we might regard *all* unmet needs as necessarily indicating an educational need. This is certainly not the case, and indeed the more skilled we become at practising dentistry and communicating with our patients, the more needs we tend to uncover. We must then decide which needs to prioritise.

Because they are usually restricted to the consultation and therefore do not formally take into account the other areas of our work, PUNs & DENs should not be relied on alone but should be part of a broader strategy to identify our learning needs. Such an approach could look at our referral patterns and our investigations, perhaps by comparing these with colleagues within the practice or the locality.

PUNs & DENs offer a snapshot view of our performance that looks quite widely but relatively superficially at what we do, and this can be complemented by forms of evaluation such as audit, which look more deeply and over a longer timescale at our work.

The technique develops our self-awareness but may ignore the perspectives of others, such as our fellow practitioners and indeed our patients, unless we seek to obtain them. How close, we may wonder, is the correlation between what *we* perceive to be a patient need and what the patient himself thinks?

How do we use PUNs & DENs in our consultations?

Identifying PUNs

Despite the limitations mentioned above, the approach is both powerful and useful, so how could we go about identifying PUNs & DENs? The following represents one method.

We need to adopt an appropriate mind-set. Although we are likely to uncover many unmet needs, this does not mean that we are necessarily bad or negligent dentists – just honest ones!

Especially in the early days, we should ensure that our experience of this technique is a positive one. As well as PUNs, there will be many PAMs – *P*atient's *A*ctually *M*et needs (apologies to Dr Eve) – and we should recognise these and pat ourselves on the back for them.

The approach requires us to think about the content of the consultation as soon after the interaction as possible. In particular, we should think about the presenting complaint, any hidden agenda, and the patient's ideas, concerns and expectations regarding the consultation. We should consider to what extent we determined any or all of these by, for example, asking ourselves whether we enquired of the patient what *his* thoughts were? Because we principally provide a technical service within many consultations, we may feel that these considerations are irrelevant. However, we are treating a person, not simply a set of teeth, and we only have to look at the complaints that are received in practice to recognise that many of them could have been avoided if the patient's concerns and understanding were explored rather than assumed.

Next, we need to consider which management options were arrived at and whether we shared these with the patient. If we did, the patient may have voiced a preference for the problem to be managed in a particular way and we should consider whether this wish was respected, and if not, for what reasons. Might it have been that we lacked the ability to implement a particular option? If so, an educational need may have been demonstrated.

Sometimes we are only aware that a PUN might have been present because the outcome of the consultation was unsatisfactory, with one or both parties feeling dissatisfied. Dissatisfaction is a sign that a need has not been met and that there are lessons to be learned by reflecting on this. The process of reflection is time-consuming and therefore this needs to be allowed for. If we don't put time aside for reflection, it simply will not happen.

Making a record

Having identified the PUNs, we need to make a record. Several examples are shown below along with guidelines to help us complete the proforma. A blank proforma that you can use can be found at the end of this chapter.

Consultation

Make a one-line note to remind ourselves of the consultation and its circumstances (remember we may not be analysing and acting on this information for a little while).

PUNs

On reflection, which PUNs did we identify? We need to be as precise as possible, framing PUNs in such a way as to make it easier to translate them into specific educational needs. It is preferable, especially when new to this technique, not to overlook any PUNs, for reasons explained below.

Why were the needs unmet?

Make a note of our thoughts. Remember that this is a record made by ourselves *for* ourselves, so we can afford to be honest. Such honesty is important because it helps us to decide why certain PUNs occurred and therefore how significant they are.

It is helpful to think about the reasons in terms of deficiencies in *knowledge, skills, attitudes* and *resources.* To illustrate this let us consider two examples from paediatric dentistry. First, suppose that a nine-year-old child presented

Table 6.1: PUNs & DENs analysis sheet

No.	Consultation details	PUNs identified	Why were the needs unmet?	DENs – what deficiencies have you identified?	Action
1	Patient attended with loose abutment screw on implant-retained prosthesis.	Patient needed reliable retention of their implant prosthesis.	I didn't know how to prevent a recurrence of the problem.	Do I know how to make an appropriate case selection? Should I use superior high torque screws? Should I change my implant system?	Talk to colleagues, manufacturers and laboratories. Consider purchasing new system?
2	Patient attended with acute abscess following re-root-treatment of tooth with chronic apical infection.	Patient needed this condition managing without precipitating acute episode.	I didn't know why this had happened.	I need to update my knowledge of re-root-treatment.	Attend course. (The course revealed that chronic conditions are associated with *E. faecalis* resistant to conventional CaOH treatment – use iodine!)
3	Patient attended requiring implants in the anterior maxillae. These could not be provided due to atrophic ridge.	I cannot do the implants because patient didn't want referral for an additional graft procedure.	I cannot carry out the ridge expansion technique, which would avoid grafting.	Lack of training and equipment to effect ridge expansion.	Attend course Buy equipment if I decide to go ahead.

with an avulsed central incisor tooth. We may not meet her need for the best treatment for this condition because of a lack of:

- *knowledge* of the most appropriate treatment
- *skill* in applying a flexible wire orthodontic splint.

Second, suppose a child presented with a decayed deciduous tooth. We may not give the appropriate treatment because of our lack of:

- an appropriate *attitude*, perhaps believing the condition to be relatively unimportant
- *resources*, in that we are running late and haven't the time to investigate further.

DENs

Now look at the PUNs and the reasons for them, as we should be able to categorise our deficiency in the manner shown above by using this information. Resources were mentioned because it is important to know when needs cannot be met through further dental education alone.

Next, we should write down how the deficiency we have identified could be corrected. We needn't worry at this stage about *precisely* how it could be done as that is the purpose of our personal development plan, but instead we should state our learning needs in general terms.

Some deficiencies are easy to identify. For example, for the child with a traumatised tooth we may write, 'I feel unsure about this topic and I need to find out what the most appropriate approach would be in this situation'.

Some deficiencies are more difficult to correct, due to an attitudinal problem that we may have. For instance, in the example of the child with a decayed deciduous tooth we may have regarded the patient's problem as being unimportant. We may have written, 'My problem is to do with my attitude towards this condition. I need to think about *why* I haven't felt uncomfortable enough about it to change my management.'

Such reflection is useful as we may find that we feel that treating the tooth is futile because the tooth would be lost anyway. We may feel that treating children is difficult and stressful or that the remuneration for any restorative treatment is prohibitively low. We could then decide whether any of these factors could or should be corrected.

Recognising that children suffer if abscesses develop (with the possible additional risk of a general anaesthetic), or that precious space might be lost for the permanent successor tooth, might help to change our attitude and therefore our behaviour.

It was mentioned that we should not *ignore* the unmet needs that we disclose. This is because over a series of consultations we may find that the same, seemingly unimportant, unmet needs keep recurring. Here are two examples.

Suppose that we discovered over the course of time that we usually failed to provide oral hygiene instruction. Thinking about this, we might discover that this was due to a lack of time and a lack of motivation. Having identified the need, we might decide to delegate this task to the dental nurse and to send her on an oral health education course so that, in future, patients could be made aware of their periodontal status and how to maintain their oral health.

In the second example, we might find that we continually felt uneasy about worn dentition because of our uncertainty about how to tackle the problem. This may make us define an educational need such as learning how to recognise occlusal disharmonies.

Action

Having decided on our educational need, the next task is to determine how to address it. For this, we need to write down the *initial* step that we intend to take. The purpose of the 'action' box is not to define exactly how the educational need will be met but rather to act as a catalyst to ensure that progress occurs. To this end it is important that our first step is feasible given the resources that are available, and that the timescale is one which we know can be achieved. Once these targets have been set, achieving them forms part of our PDP, for which we need to think about how we can demonstrate to ourselves and to others that our needs have been met and that our behaviour has changed.

At its most basic level, this evidence may come from observing our future PUNs & DENs – do they confirm that the same unmet needs do not keep recurring? More sophisticated evidence of learning may be in the form of teaching others, writing a guideline or protocol, or conducting an audit. This should not put us off, however, as committing ourselves to do no more than just *think* about what we have learned is a very good place to start.

Inviting others to contribute to our PUNs & DENs exercise is not mandatory, but can greatly increase its value. Asking a colleague to consider our activity by looking at our PUNs and DENs analysis sheet and hearing our thoughts about it gives us the opportunity to gain a different perspective and hopefully a greater insight into our skills. Such colleagues may also be able to help us to improve our skills. Most dentists regard such an invitation to contribute as a privilege, and links established in this way can improve relationships greatly. Who knows, you may be asked to return the favour!

How could the practice team use PUNs & DENs?

Determining PUNs & DENs not only helps the individual to recognise his strengths and weaknesses, but also, if the information is shared, helps a team to build up a profile of the range of knowledge and skills possessed by its members. Using such a profile, priorities for education can be set because when an educational deficiency is common to several members of the team, then a *Team Educational Need* (a *TEN* rather than a *DEN*) has been demonstrated.

☑ **Checkpoint 6.1**

As an example, suppose that the dentists in the practice recognised that they shared a common PUN, namely that although patients often asked about aesthetic dentistry options, they were not given advice about them. Discussion of the matter might reveal that this was because dentists regarded the time taken to give advice as leading to a perceived loss of earnings.

Discussion within the team might then lead to possible solutions, such as training a receptionist to offer the appropriate advice or producing patient information leaflets. What previously was thought to be a money-losing activity could then become an income-generating one.

The PUNs & DENs of the team could also be determined by conducting other types of evaluation. For example, an audit of clinical care or of patient complaints may highlight differences between partners from which PUNs could be inferred and DENs derived.

When individuals undertake their own PUNs & DENs exercise, they obtain comments from their colleagues only if these are requested. If the *team* uses the technique in the way described it is vital that the individuals assessed are handled sensitively both with regard to how deficiencies are exposed and how these might be remedied. One approach is to use the method described for team-based feedback in Chapter 7 on significant event analysis.

Just as dentists have to make arrangements to attend to their DENs, if a TEN is present it may be worthwhile and cost-effective to arrange for group tuition. 'Educational resources' usually means people with particular knowledge, *experience* or skills, and such resources could be shared on a reciprocal arrangement between teams.

The word 'experience' is highlighted because this is something we *all* acquire from the earliest stages of our careers. People who have experience are often the best teachers, as they know immediately what the difficulties are and how best to overcome them. Looked at in this way, many people within the team are potential teachers as well as practitioners, and good ones at that.

Summary

As we can see, the PUNs & DENs approach is an extremely practical one. In our own ways, we use it frequently but never glorify it with a title! So much for the theory. The proforma overleaf is simple to use and dovetails easily with your PDP, so why not photocopy it and give it a try?

PUNs & DENs: analysis sheet

No.	Consultation details	PUNs identified	Why were the needs unmet?	DENs – what deficiencies have you identified?	Action
1					
2					
3					

7 Significant event analysis (SEA)

What is SEA?

What's in a name?

How can SEA help us?

What types of significant event are there?

How can we conduct a SEA?

Significant event examples and analysis sheets

Using significant events in the PDP

Summary

Further information

Key points

- Significant events in our professional lives can be examples of when things go significantly right as well as significantly wrong.
- They can be analysed through individual reflection or in larger groups.
- Discussing them with the practice team allows whole-patient care across the team to be assessed.
- The outcomes of SEA include celebration or the recognition of good practice, as well as the demonstration of a need for audit or for an immediate change in behaviour.
- Significant events can be used systematically to study particular areas of our service.
- These areas may be organisational as well as clinical.

- There are some ground rules for the way in which significant events are discussed, which maximise the benefits of the process.
- Keeping records allows the team to learn and individuals to use the experience in forming their PDPs.

What is SEA?

Of the many events that happen to and around us in practice life, significant events are those which make an impact on the mind (and the heart). They can be examples of when things go significantly *right* as well as significantly wrong and can be clinical or non-clinical events, involving anyone from one person to the entire team. Because *we* regard them as significant, they are powerful motivators for change, and this can be harnessed through the process of significant event analysis (SEA).

SEA is the mechanism by which we look at noteworthy events in our practice lives with the purpose of learning from and celebrating good practice as well as improving suboptimal practice. Experience shows that the great benefit which people derive from SEA is out of proportion to the effort it requires.

What's in a name?

SEA seems to go by various names: significant event audit, critical event audit or analysis, significant event review and so on.

The term 'significant event' has been chosen because the term 'critical' implies incidents which are negative in their consequences, which, as we have said, is not always so. The word 'analysis' has been used because this term is broad-ranging and does not commit us to undertaking an audit cycle.

How can SEA help us?

Let us illustrate this with an example. Suppose that a patient collapsed during dental treatment.

We could look at this incident to determine whether there are any lessons to be learned, by asking ourselves the following questions.

- What went well?
- What went badly?
- How could I improve?

The answer to the last question might identify a learning need that we could use in our PDP.

This simple analysis could be done quickly, perhaps in discussion with a colleague, and would involve a minimum of paperwork. However, we could go one step further and discuss the same incident with our teams, thus using the full potential of SEA to assess the quality of service delivered by *all* those involved in the patient's care. The sort of questions that might be asked of different team members and services are illustrated below.

Dentists

- Was the alarm raised?
- Did the dentist maintain the airway and provide basic cardiopulmonary resuscitation (CPR)?
- Did the dentist have a defibrillator, and if so, did he know when and how to use it?

Dental nurse

- Did the dental nurse get the oxygen (the availability of which is a service requirement)?
- Did the nurse bring the emergency drugs?

Receptionists

- Did the receptionist phone for an ambulance and give a minimum data set (e.g. age/status/address/nature of problem)?
- Did the receptionist request an immediate response?

Ambulance services

- Was there any difficulty contacting the service?
- Was the response time adequate?

Other issues

- After the event: were the drugs in date and when was the oxygen last checked?
- Were the spanner to open the oxygen supply and the connecting tubes readily available?

This list is not intended to be exhaustive, but it gives an idea of the range of disciplines involved in a single significant event. It also demonstrates our interdependence and the fact that good-quality care requires competence at *all* levels.

Performing a SEA using this incident could lead to one of four outcomes.

The need for immediate change

Suppose that it came to light that the patient had a history of reaction to local anaesthetic, but that this had not been recorded prominently in the notes. The practice would need to correct this immediately and to ensure that a system was put in place for routinely warning dentists about allergies/adverse reactions and other risk factors prior to treatment.

Demonstration of the need for an audit

Perhaps the dentist did not feel comfortable about performing modern CPR. A brief audit of other dentists and nurses within the practice, looking at when they were last formally updated on CPR skills, might reveal a need for retraining.

Recognition of good practice

Whereby all that could have been done, had been done. The team could feel justifiably proud of attaining high standards in the knowledge that although this awful event happened, it could not have been prevented.

Celebration

Although this sounds incongruous, celebration may be justified where exemplary care is seen. For example, the dentist might have appropriately used a defibrillator even though most other practices in the area did not have one.

Because SEA looks at the performance of several people, it is possible that more than one outcome will be seen. Thus some individuals or groups will see their actions vindicated or praised, while others will acknowledge that there is work to be done. The way in which feedback is given is therefore highly important if the team as a whole is not to be divided.

As we can see, even if we thought that the significant event did not involve us directly, attending a SEA meeting may make us look at our actions and thereby bring to light learning needs of which we were previously unaware.

☑ **Checkpoint 7.1**

Can you think of a significant event within your own practice that involved members of the team other than yourself? Write down the first that springs to mind.

Now think about the barriers to using SEA in relation to this event. What are these?

☑ **Checkpoint 7.1 discussion**

You will have seen that identifying significant events is not difficult – they are all about us and they are usually memorable. Hopefully, you will have identified an event that has implications beyond your own personal responsibility and you will have recognised that talking about it could prove challenging.

Here are some of the common barriers to using significant events:

* admitting that we make mistakes

- concerns over confidentiality – how will we know that our mistakes will not be publicised?
- the fear that we might lose the esteem or confidence of our colleagues
- knowing how to use significant events in a positive way
- having the opportunity to do so.

What types of significant event are there?

We define events as being significant because they are thought to be important in our professional lives or the life of the practice, or because they may offer some insight into the standards of care that the practice provides. Most people start with events that are dramatic by virtue of their nature or consequences, and use these to learn from. Here are some examples.

1 A vocational dental practitioner suffers a needle-stick injury and finds that there is no experienced practitioner available to speak to who might advise him as to what action to take.

2 A patient suffers persistent anaesthesia lasting for several months following trauma to the inferior dental nerve after removal of a lower third molar.

3 A complaint regarding breach of confidentiality follows an incident in which a patient was asked at the receptionist's desk if she was pregnant. This question was asked in order to determine whether the patient was exempt from dental charges.

☑ **Checkpoint 7.2**

Having read these examples, make a note below of the issues for the practice that might arise from these three significant events.

1

2

3

☑ **Checkpoint 7.2 discussion**

1 In the first example, the issues might be as follows.

- Should a vocational practitioner be left unsupervised?
- Are systems in place for contacting a more experienced colleague? What are the vocational practitioner's educational needs regarding this event?
- Does the practice need a protocol to provide guidance on needle-stick injuries?
- Who else, e.g. dental nurses, needs to be updated on the management of such injuries?

2 In the second example, issues of clinical skills and consent arise.

- There is a need for careful pre-operative radiographic assessment to check the proximity of the apex to the inferior dental nerve. Was this done?
- Did the dentist obtain proper informed consent prior to the procedure? Was there a record of this in the notes?

3 The third example illustrates the ease with which confidentiality might unintentionally be broken.

- Does the receptionist understand the importance of confidentiality and the implications if it is breached?
- Do patients know why certain questions might be asked?
- Can the practice obtain the information it requires in other ways, e.g. by using a questionnaire?
- Does the practice have facilities (for example, a private room) where sensitive questions can be asked?
- Could the design of the reception area be improved in order to reduce the risk?

We can learn from significant events as they arise, in which case the areas of personal and practice activity that we end up examining in detail are a matter of chance. There is nothing wrong in doing this. When starting from scratch, it is important not to make the SEA too complicated and it is far better to have a simple approach that is quickly adopted and found useful than to have one that is too involved.

When we have more experience with SEA, another approach is to keep a record of significant events when they occur, and categorise them according to the area of activity into which they fall. We can then audit our service systematically by choosing an area and analysing the event associated with it. This approach is sometimes called significant event audit.

Examples of these areas are:

- clinical: preventive, acute and chronic
- organisational

Let us now consider these areas in more detail with some examples of significant events in each and how they could be used.

Clinical: preventive care

A six-year-old child who presents with occlusal caries

This might represent a breakdown in oral hygiene care. Here are some issues raised by this event.

- Was there an assessment of caries susceptibility in this child? In the records, we might look specifically for a record of the number of cavities in the deciduous teeth, which might have prompted the use of fissure sealants on the first permanent molars.
- Was appropriate dietary counselling given?
- Was oral hygiene instruction given to both child and parent? If we can't tell, this would raise issues of appropriate record keeping as well as clinical care.

Other examples of significant events in preventive care: *failure to give advice about fluoride, or failure to diagnose enamel/dentine maturation anomalies.*

If significant events were found to be rare, then significant event audit would have the effect of showing that high standards of preventive care are being achieved.

Clinical: acute care

Serious diagnosis: oral cancer

A new cancer diagnosis prompts us to review the patient records and ask the following questions.

- When was the condition first diagnosed?
- When did the patient first present with symptoms which in retrospect might have been attributable to the condition?
- Could we reasonably say that the condition should have been suspected at an earlier stage?
- When was the patient referred – should this have been done sooner?
- How quickly was the patient seen after referral – was this acceptable?

It may well be that the patient was examined at the first presentation, referred and seen urgently and hence no delay occurred.

Missed diagnosis

Everyone misses diagnoses; the important thing is recognising the fact and learning from our mistakes. Here are a few real-life examples.

- *Failure to diagnose acid erosion in a bulimic patient.* This would remind us to examine more closely – for example, looking for cupping of the molar cusps or thinning and breakdown of the incisor edges.
- *Persistent oral pain in a menopausal woman, unresponsive to dental intervention.* The cause might be 'burning mouth syndrome', recognition of which would prevent misdiagnosis as chronic atrophic candidosis and the use of inappropriate antifungal treatment.
- *Failure to spot potential premalignant lesions* – due to the examiner's fixation on dental hard tissue!

These are diagnoses which we could or should have made, but failed to make. These diagnoses usually come to light when another colleague is involved and this raises two additional points.

First, while we are ready to involve another professional (usually a specialist and therefore not a peer) when we are having clinical difficulties, we are less willing to see our deficiencies uncovered by our practice colleagues or indeed by our patients.

Being 'exposed' in this way may amount to no more than seeing an entry in the clinical records when another dentist has been involved in the patient's care, or getting some friendly feedback from a colleague over a cup of coffee. Sometimes our patients prompt us with an article from a newspaper about a condition that seems to fit their symptoms. Although it is hard at the time to see it this way, these incidents are opportunities for education and improvement even though they may initially feel like unwelcome or presumptious criticism.

Second, it is important that colleagues who uncover such missed diagnoses take the opportunity to let the relevant parties learn from the incident while exercising sensitivity over the manner and forum in which they do so.

Clinical: chronic dental conditions

Loss of teeth secondary to failed periodontal monitoring

Suppose that a solicitor's letter claims that failure to diagnose, treat or refer appropriately has led to the patient losing their teeth. This might raise issues such as the following.

- Were appropriate radiographs taken?
- Was basic periodontal evaluation (BPE) undertaken?
- If BPE scores were high, did the dentist perform an in-depth evaluation to consider complex treatment or referral?

Secondary caries in complex crown and bridge work

A patient with complex crown and bridge work requires this to be replaced because of secondary caries. We know that instead of 'fitting and forgetting', dentists should adopt a 'fit and maintain approach'.

- Was BPE performed to monitor dental health?
- Was the patient shown (not just told) how to perform effective interdental cleaning?
- Was routine radiographic surveillance performed to reflect the caries susceptibility of the individual?

- Was there a good call and recall system to ensure that the patient was monitored regularly?

Other examples of significant events in chronic care: *destabilising occlusion, secondary to the failure to correct tooth substance loss. Denture-induced hyperplasia (false ridges), secondary to the failure to reduce overextended flanges on the dentures as the alveolus resorbs. Angular cheilitis, secondary to failure to maintain the correct vertical face height on the denture.*

Organisational

This heading covers a multitude of sins – and successes! Significant events can occur in many non-clinical domains of practice life so let us look at some examples in each area.

Service delivery

An important route by which shortcomings in the delivery of care can be highlighted is the patient complaint. We have always taken complaints seriously and nowadays there is a contractual duty to deal with them in a professional manner. However, this duty does not require us to discuss the lessons learned but merely to report that the process has been observed and that the outcome has, or has not, been successful.

Patient complaints can highlight aspects of the quality, range and accessibility of both our clinical and non-clinical services. As partners in healthcare, patients are increasingly being encouraged to contribute and their suggestions for improvement as well as their positive feedback regarding our services could be used as significant events from which to learn.

Practice management

- *Problems with protocols*: these seem to become ever more prolific, but nevertheless remain necessary. For example, the lack of implementation of a protocol for ensuring the optimum processing of films can lead to a reduced diagnostic yield. This would raise issues concerning the processing of films – for example, how often the x-ray developer fluid is changed as well as how films should be labelled and stored.

- *Staff management*: significant events may arise as a result of mistakes, sometimes brought to light through the feedback or complaints of patients or through the routine supervision of practice activity. This may highlight training issues, but the areas of performance review, employment law and disciplinary action may also need to be considered. Staff may themselves be upset by the behaviour of the patients or, dare it be said, the dentists themselves, thus creating other issues which need to be addressed.

  We should not forget that there are numerous examples relating to staff in which difficult situations are managed particularly well by individuals or groups. These significant events should be used as opportunities to demonstrate to them that their efforts are noticed and appreciated by their colleagues. Such tokens of recognition are often valued more by individuals than the financial rewards of their work.

- *Financial management*: good dental practice can only be maintained if income is efficiently generated. For obvious reasons, significant events relating to financial management usually generate immediate responses! Here are two examples.

  - Payment confusion may arise and income lost if the claim mechanism is not clearly identified – for example, if it is not clearly stated whether payment is to be made on completion of treatment or in instalments during the treatment programme.

  - Fees may be lost if record cards have been misfiled and as a result claim forms have not been sent to the Dental Practice Board (DPB), or if the DPB schedules have not been routinely checked.

- *Estate management*: by which I mean attending to the practice building and contents. Water damage may force us to attend to the upkeep of the dental surgery roof, and a burglary might prompt a review of the security arrangements and insurance cover.

  Less dramatic events can be studied in order to prevent future disasters. For example, an electric heater left on overnight might just be considered to be a disciplinary matter. However, used as a significant event, it could encourage the practice to review the fire regulations for public buildings, to invite the local fire officer to inspect the building and make recommendations, and to ensure that the practice staff undertake a periodic fire drill.

How can we conduct a SEA?

The key point here is that SEA should be felt to be a positive experience by those involved in it. The fact that we are engaging in the process at all is itself commendable and this should be applauded.

Who is going to be involved, when and where?

Most significant events involve several people in the team and it is usually appropriate for those concerned to discuss and learn from the experience together. Dentists and dental nurses are increasingly encouraged to set time aside for professional development. However, SEA may require the attendance of other employees (for example, the receptionists, practice manager or dental hygienist) and protected time will have to be arranged. Note that the implication is that dentists or nurses make the decision as to which events will be discussed and in what sort of forum. As practice teams develop it is hoped that other members, such as employees, will be similarly empowered.

How soon after a significant event should it be analysed? This depends largely on the event, with those that may indicate a serious shortcoming requiring immediate attention. With other events it is useful to have time to reflect on matters before formally conducting a SEA, but the length of time should not be too great otherwise momentum will be lost and details forgotten. Hence details of a significant event should be recorded as soon as we become aware that one has taken place.

Getting into the habit of routinely conducting SEA means that any anxiety associated with the process is reduced and the experience becomes more influential in shaping our future behaviour.

SEA is not just an uncovering of facts and the formulation of action points – there are sometimes strong feelings involved and it is important that the group is not interrupted from without or within (mobile phones and bleeps). You may wish to consider which environment is the most conducive. Meetings outside the workplace are more likely to encourage people to open up, but may be less convenient and less focused on problem solving.

What are the ground rules?

SEA requires participants to be honest with each other. Those involved must feel that they have entered into the process willingly and are both prepared to play an active part and to learn from the experience. Confidentiality should not be assumed but should be made explicit and some clear guidelines should be established as to what could be discussed outside the group.

So how do you get it right? One approach is to ask others who have conducted SEA to advise you, or even help you by facilitating a meeting. In return, as your experience develops you may be able to offer a similar service to others. Just as dentists can collaborate educationally, so practices can provide co-facilitation.

Even if a facilitator is not used, meetings of more than four people generally need a chairperson to make sure that all those present have a chance to contribute, that conflict does not escalate and that appropriate records are kept. These records are usually a note of the significant event itself, what went well, what went badly and, as a result of discussion, what recommendations are being made for improvement.

Let us now consider the key stages in conducting a SEA. The process is described for a significant event with negative connotations, only because these are the types most often discussed. When positive events are analysed, not all the points made below will be relevant.

Why has this significant event been chosen?

It is useful to establish why this event is significant and to determine what those involved wish to achieve by analysing it. Sometimes the process starts with an individual who feels unhappy, perhaps guilty, about an event and wishes to explore it further, in which case the purpose of SEA is partly to address the need of the individual. At other times personal feelings may not be involved but there may be an issue of practice performance that needs to be addressed collectively.

What are the facts of the case?

To save time it is useful to circulate the factual material relating to the event prior to the meeting, such as the date and time, nature of the event, the circumstances and the people involved. Those principally involved will need to have done some background work, perhaps by reviewing the patient records or establishing the sequence of events. In addition, they should be prepared to talk about how the event was managed and whether there are, or might be, longer-term consequences.

For many significant events the only 'props' needed for SEA are the patient records, but any relevant material should be brought to the meeting.

What issues are raised?

Having clarified the facts, the next stage is to decide what issues are raised by the event. We will want to consider each of these issues in turn in order to decide if any action is needed. To illustrate this, consider the example given earlier regarding the patient who collapsed following dental treatment. We could list some of the issues as follows:

- emergency clinical care – was the treatment given by the dentist and nurse adequate?
- communication – how well did we respond to an emergency, obtain help and deal with other patients?
- equipment – were the drugs and CPR equipment immediately available?

What went well?

With these issues in mind, those involved should discuss the areas relating to the event that they feel generally positive about. This helps to put the event into perspective and, once they have spoken, others in the group should be encouraged to voice their observations of the examples of good practice that the event demonstrates – and there are *always* some.

What went badly and how could we improve?

What was it exactly that went wrong? It is important to be specific, as this helps to differentiate significant lapses in performance from the 'feel bad' surrounding the event. To achieve this, the key members should be given time to go through the following stages.

1 Talk about what went wrong.

2 Discuss their feelings with respect to the event itself.

3 Describe how they might have done things differently.

4 Discuss what they might have needed in order to do things differently in terms of knowledge, skills and resources. This step highlights areas for possible action.

5 *Invite* others in the group to make their comments. I emphasise the word invite because if the key members are encouraged to retain control at this point, their feelings of vulnerability will be reduced and they will be more likely to take note of the comments made.

Those invited, and it may be a general invitation to the whole group, could proceed along the following lines.

1 Select the major shortcoming that they perceive. Because the purpose of feedback is to improve future performance, this shortcoming should relate to a specific skill or ability that is amenable to improvement rather than one that is not, such as the colleague's personality.

2 Point out any alternative strategy that may have prevented the problem or allowed it to have been more effectively managed.

3 Highlight any skills or resources that may be needed by the person concerned to enact the suggested strategy in future.

4 Make their final comments positive ones, perhaps by reiterating what the colleague has done well, and thus encouraging him to improve. This step is important because people tend to remember the last thing that someone has said to them.

This stage of SEA would need modification if we were talking with groups of people who were jointly involved in a significant event. Personal sensibilities may not be such an issue and time constraints may not allow *individuals* to go through all the steps listed above.

Which improvements are feasible?

Having heard the deliberations of the group it is useful to summarise the key points of what went wrong and the suggestions made for improvement. We now have to decide on the appropriate action by determining which of the suggestions made are feasible, and which of these should be prioritised. This approach is a practical one which recognises that not all the factors that contribute to a problem can be remedied.

What action should be taken?

Action may involve formulating a plan based on one or more steps from the following scheme.

1 Decide which improvements are to be prioritised.
2 Determine which new skills or resources are needed to meet these requirements.
3 Plan for these needs to be met.
4 Decide on a timescale over which the improvements are to be made.
5 Consider whether and how to widen the educational benefit gained by the participants in this SEA, bearing in mind confidentiality issues and the need to anonymise data. For example, should the event be discussed in a peer-review group?
6 Consider how the success of this action plan could be determined. Are there elements in the suggested improvements that can be measured and therefore audited?

What records should we keep?

Overwhelmed as we are by paperwork it is tempting to avoid the written word when we can. With SEA this is almost always a mistake. Making a record offers the following advantages.

- Writing down the circumstances of the event helps to clarify the facts and avoid misunderstanding.
- A record can be made of the analysis itself and what action was taken as a result. This can serve as a useful summary of why things went wrong and the lessons that were learned. In the future, faced with similar circumstances, this information could prove valuable.

- Appropriate details from the record can be shared in a suitable form with a wider audience, e.g. specific details can be fed back to a patient who made a complaint. Additionally, anonymised information can be given to colleagues outside the practice who wish to learn from our experience or to organisations that require confirmation that we are undertaking such reviews.
- The process of SEA is a form of adult learning. Making a record of the deliberations could allow the time spent to be accredited as part of our PDP.

Significant event examples and analysis sheets

The practice could decide what the record should contain, but three examples of the sort of record that could be kept are shown below.

The first is an abbreviated record such as could be kept to note the main outcomes of a SEA meeting. The second and third are examples of a more detailed record which individuals could complete for their PDPs. This record is in two sections – the first uses questions that encourage reflection on the significant event, and the second uses questions that help us to plan our learning.

Examples demonstrating how the analysis sheets could be completed are given, followed by blank sheets for your own use.

Significant event: Saturday morning emergency surgery – patient behaved in an aggressive manner toward the receptionist

Issues arising from discussion	• Staff safety • Security of premises • Panic buttons • Removal of patients from the list
Positive points	• Patient was calmed down by receptionist • On-call dentist was alerted without inflaming the situation • Patient was recognised as being ill (schizophrenic) and *not* subsequently removed from the list of registered patients • The patient's medical practitioner was informed
Concerns	• Potential for harm: receptionist was on her own, waiting room was otherwise empty • Patient was able to lean across into the reception area • There was no panic button to call for help
Suggestions	• Redesign reception counter • Install panic buttons • Consider staff training • Ask the advice of the local police
Action	• Training session organised for the team regarding how to manage potentially violent patients • Arrange quotes for new fixtures • Apply for grant for this equipment • Ensure that phones in the reception area have a direct dial to the police station

Significant event analysis sheet: example 1

Reflection

1 Description of the event
  • A patient presented as an emergency with a painful tooth. The event was the creation of an oro-antral fistula (OAF) during the extraction of an upper first permanent molar tooth. Tooth decoronated during a forceps extraction. The roots were divided with an oral surgery fissure bur during which the antrum was perforated.

2 Issues raised by the event
  • An inadequate pre-operative radiograph failed to warn of the proximity of the antrum.
  • Inadequate time was allowed for the procedure resulting in an excessive amount of tissue loss.
  • There was no pre-operative counselling of the patient.

3 What went well
  • The extraction was completed.
  • The fistula was diagnosed and the patient informed.
  • Appropriate post-operative management was used and the patient was reviewed.
  • An early oral surgery referral was made.

4 What didn't go well
  • The pre-operative assessment was poor.
  • Procedure was hurried.
  • Because of the extensive tissue loss, the first oral surgery repair was unsuccessful.
  • A second repair was required and this necessitated a bone graft.

5 How I might have done things differently
  • A more careful pre-operative assessment would have disclosed the patient's history of chronic sinusitis. This would have alerted me to the possibility of an enlarged antrum.

- The patient was a fit-in. I was hurried and used an inadequate radiograph. On reflection, I should have taken another film.
- I should have given adequate pre-operative counselling to warn of the possibility of a fistula.
- I was rushed. I should have made a decision to carry out the procedure electively, perhaps later in the day when I had more time.

Significant event analysis sheet: example 1

Action

6 Areas of feasible improvement

- Ensure that I make an adequate risk assessment of the possibility of creating a fistula.
- Specifically, make sure that I never proceed with an operative procedure without an adequate pre-operative radiograph.
- Ensure that I give routine pre-operative counselling where there is a significant possibility of complications.

7 Educational needs identified

- Revise my radiographic technique, specifically so that when I take a PA view, I can see the crown, roots and associated structures and avoid coning.
- Learn how to perform an adequate risk assessment.
- Learn how to remove roots in a way that minimises the possibility of creating an OAF.

8 Which needs I will address and in what order

- In the order stated above. This is because an adequate radiograph is critical to the risk assessment. Proper risk assessment would allow me to refer patients for appropriate surgery rather than attempt the procedure myself.

9 How I intend to meet those needs

- Revising from the radiographic textbooks/talking to colleagues.
- Attend an appropriate hands-on minor surgery course.

10 How I will be able to demonstrate improvement

- Audit my PA radiographs, looking to see that all relevant structures are clearly visible.
- Audit my root extractions, looking for the complication rate before and after attendance at the hands-on minor surgery course.

Significant event analysis sheet: example 2

Reflection

1 Description of the event

- The mother of a patient complained in the reception area that the practice was responsible for her son being hospitalised and close to death. The son had a valvular lesion, had received fissure sealant and a scaling treatment from the dental hygienist and had subsequently developed infective endocarditis.

2 Issues raised by the event

- Are we clear about those conditions that require antibiotic cover?
- Did we know about the valvular lesion? Were we taking an adequate medical history and updating this regularly?
- Did we advise the patient to take antibiotics and did we issue a prescription?
- Was the patient given appropriate advice to take antibiotics within one hour of the planned treatment?
- Was the practice forewarned that the patient coming in for treatment needed antibiotic cover?
- Did we confirm that the patient had taken the antibiotic cover appropriately?
- Is a dental hygienist the appropriate person to treat a patient who is at risk of endocarditis?

3 What went well

- We had a system that worked to a degree.
- We knew the indications for antibiotic cover, recognised the need in this patient and issued an appropriate prescription.
- We knew that the patient was coming in for treatment under antibiotic cover and asked if he had taken the medication.
- The last two facts are known because of reasonable record keeping.

4 What didn't go well

- Although we asked if antibiotics had been taken, we have no record of the time at which the antibiotics were taken in relation to the treatment given.
- We knew that the patient was at risk, but we had no way of demonstrating that appropriate questions about endocarditis risk were asked at the appropriate times.

5 How I might have done things differently

- I would have ensured that the records were clearly marked regarding endocarditis risk.
- I would have recorded how long before treatment the patient had taken the antibiotics.

Significant event analysis sheet: example 2

Action

6 Areas of feasible improvement

- Record risk, ensuring that this is done systematically and repeatedly. Use a sticker system with a sticker being placed on the most recent dental record.
- Develop a protocol for identifying at-risk patients, confirming at-risk status with general medical practitioner, prescribing appropriate antibiotic, alerting practice prior to attendance for treatment, recording patient compliance and the time at which antibiotic was taken.
- Altering our dental management, so that patients who require procedures under antibiotic cover are treated by a dentist rather than by a hygienist.

7 Educational needs identified

- Know the indications for antibiotic cover.
- Know the appropriate procedure for taking antibiotics prior to dental treatment.
- Know how best to check for compliance.

8 Which needs I will address and in what order

- All of the above.

9 How I intend to meet those needs

- Look at the guidelines in the *British National Formulary.*
- Contact the local dental tutor.
- Discuss with a cardiac physician.

10 How I will be able to demonstrate improvement

- Produce the new protocol for antibiotic cover.
- Audit patient records: looking to see that the new risk-factor sticker has been put on the most recent dental record and, where present, has been completed.

Significant event analysis sheet: team example

Reflection

1 Description of the event

2 Issues raised by the event

3 What went well

4 What didn't go well

5 How I might have done things differently

Significant event analysis sheet: team example

Action

6   Areas of feasible improvement

7   Educational needs identified

8   Which needs I will address and in what order

9   How I intend to meet those needs

10   How I will be able to demonstrate improvement

Using significant events in the PDP

Once we become adept at thinking in terms of significant events and how they might be used, it becomes a simple matter to incorporate them in our PDPs. We have seen how they can be studied in depth and this analysis can help us to take the emotion out of the situation and to recognise our learning needs.

As we become practised with this technique, we may choose not to fill in a significant event analysis sheet but simply to translate these events directly into educational needs and objectives. This is illustrated in Table 7.1 with an endodontic example using the PDP layout with which you are now familiar.

☑ **Checkpoint 7.3**

In Table 7.2, use a significant event of your own to complete the shaded box. Following this, complete the adjacent boxes, identifying the educational need which you feel is the most important and then writing out one or two specific objectives in relation to this.

Summary

Most dentists can't help talking about their work. It fascinates us, and we are often keen to share anything that is out of the ordinary with our colleagues. We also seem to instinctively realise that significant events are a rich vein from which to extract our learning. Capturing and making constructive use of this fascination with the unusual is the essence of significant event analysis. Of all the techniques discussed in this handbook, it is the one which, even in the most rudimentary form, you should make use of.

Table 7.1: Using a significant event in the PDP

Educational need	Reason for inclusion in development plan	Development objectives	Activities to be used	What evidence will you keep?
To provide more predictable success rates of endodontics using a safe technique.	A patient almost swallowed a dental file last week. I'm fed up of failed endodontic cases that result in extraction.	Be able to put on rubber dam successfully on 90% of cases within two minutes.		

Table 7.2: Using a significant event in the PDP

Educational need	Reason for inclusion in development plan	Development objectives	Activities to be used	What evidence will you keep?

Further information

Pringle M, Bradley C, Carmichael C, Wallis H and Moore A (1995) *Significant Event Auditing.* Occasional Paper No. 70. Royal College of General Practitioners, London.

This paper explains the principles of SEA in more detail, particularly the way in which SEA is used by practices to audit their care.

8 Clinical audit

Key points

■ Audit is a method by which we look systematically and critically at our work with the objective of improving patient care.

■ It can help us to identify deficiencies, encourage us to change and reduce the errors that we might make. It can also demonstrate good standards of care.

■ Audits can be performed by ourselves, in association with our colleagues or by external assessors.

■ Audit is not about 'naming and shaming', but about encouraging improvements in performance within a supportive environment.

■ The audit process involves setting standards and measuring our performance against these.

■ Making changes in order to improve our performance and then repeating the audit is the mechanism by which we complete the audit cycle.

■ Various agencies can advise as to how to engage in audit, and audit protocols are readily available.

Introduction

From a once-esoteric activity, audit is becoming more commonplace, spurred on by clinical governance directives and the changes in NHS dentists' Terms of Service regarding audit and peer review. However, audit should not be regarded as an imposition. The technique is often used for practice management, and practices that are well run, profitable and deliver high-quality care almost always incorporate audit as part of their routine activity.

Here, we are concerned with how audit can help us from an educational viewpoint and our focus will be on clinical audit activity. We will look first at the benefits of engaging in clinical audit and then go on to consider in more detail how it can be undertaken, some of the difficulties involved and how we can ensure that our efforts bear fruit. At the end of the chapter, we will see from an example of clinical audit how education, patient care and profitability are linked.

What is clinical audit?

Put simply, clinical audit is the method by which health professionals look systematically and critically at their work with the purpose of enhancing the health of their patients.

Although dentists can conduct audit on their own, to gain more value as well as more enjoyment from the process, it is best regarded as a group activity. In larger practices, dentists can band together, but single-handed practitioners will need to involve colleagues from neighbouring practices. In more recent times it is becoming recognised that the delivery of dental healthcare involves other members of the dental team and, as a result, audit activity is becoming a joint venture within practices and, indeed, between practices. One insight from this multidisciplinary approach is the extent to which one team member is dependent upon the quality of work of the others – in other words, the end product is only as good as its weakest link.

To those who have not taken part in audit before, there are some common misconceptions which serve to give it a forbidding image. Here are some things that audit is *not*.

- It is *not 'research'*. In research we are unclear what 'best practice' represents and the purpose of our activity is to try to find out. In audit, we not only know what we need to do but we are able to state how well we should be able to do it.
- An audit is *not just number crunching*. Many examples of so-called audit activity are in reality little more than data collection, often done because it has been demanded by some external agency. In clinical audit, we have ownership of the process and we decide what data to collect on the basis of what *we* are trying to study and how best to use that data to improve our standards. Done in this way, audit is far from a sterile activity.
- Audit is *not about 'naming and shaming'* – it allows those whose work is being analysed to recognise where their weaknesses lie but this is very much within an environment of support. The best audits come to nothing if it is not recognised that people need first to be acknowledged for their strengths and then encouraged and supported to make the improvements that are recommended.

How could it help me?

Some of the reasons why audit is worth engaging in are listed below.

Identifying deficiencies

Clinical audit can help to identify some of our strengths and weaknesses. Often, the subject of the audit is decided on by a group of people on the basis of the interests of the practice. We may not know at the outset whether we have an area of personal need and although the outcome of the audit may sometimes confirm our worst fears, it may also show that our best hopes regarding our performance are justified.

Sometimes we may choose to undertake an audit for personal reasons, perhaps because we suspect that we have a problem area and wish to discover whether this is the case, and if so to what degree. Audit not only allows us to identify an area that needs our attention but also provides the means, through the comparison of our performance against standards which *we* set, of measuring the improvements that we try to make.

Encouraging change

Many changes that dentists are subjected to are externally imposed, but with audit we have the opportunity to decide where the priorities lie within our practices, and hence where change is needed.

Audit requires us to look objectively at the topic being considered and learn more about it before deciding on the criteria and standards. This means that when, as a group, we try to define 'best practice', we challenge the *evidence* rather than each other's opinion. Later, when the audit is performed, the data allow comparisons to be made objectively.

Hence, audit can encourage change by increasing ownership, establishing an evidence-base and depersonalising the arguments by using informed opinion rather than impressions or vested interests to make comparisons.

Reducing errors

We have touched on one form of 'error' which audit may highlight, namely that we are not treating our patients in line with currently accepted 'best practice'. This form of error can be corrected through learning.

Quite often though, we know what we should be doing but not whether we are actually doing it. Audit is a powerful tool for showing us how diligent (or otherwise) we are at putting into practice what we have learned. In addition, when changes are made and new standards or protocols are agreed, audit is the mechanism of accountability by which team members can prove to themselves and to others that protocols are being implemented.

We have said that audit is not about apportioning blame. To succeed in producing change, audit doesn't need to publicly ascribe blame to the individual, but *does* need to allow those involved to make comparisons. Dentists often compare themselves with their peers and don't like to be seen as 'below average', and this is a powerful motivator for self-improvement. This factor should be borne in mind when audit results are discussed.

☑ **Checkpoint 8.1**

What sort of audit can expose potential clinical errors? Let us take an example.

Suppose that we conducted an audit of bite-wing radiographs. What might we learn from this?

☑ **Checkpoint 8.1 discussion**

Audit of radiographs can cover such areas as the technical aspects of film processing, but it can also look at how the radiograph was taken and the implications of this.

In this example, if our retrospective analysis of a series of radiographs showed that we were continually coning off the edge of the film, we might decide to routinely use a film holder and perform a further audit after a period of time to check that our performance had improved.

Now think about radiography within your own practice. What aspect would you audit and why?

Even simple audits like this are likely to uncover significant gaps in care, some of which may have medico-legal implications. Hence, reducing error through audit is an important way of preventing harm to the patient and of reducing the risk to ourselves.

Demonstrating good care

We might believe that our practice delivers high-quality care, but how could we prove it? Audit provides the mechanism for doing this and is a key element in the clinical governance programmes which are being introduced, as well as being part of the revalidation process.

Additionally, because audit is not a closed circle but a continuous process, new standards can be set and re-audits conducted further down the line to demonstrate that good standards are maintained and that poorer standards have been raised.

Who does the audit?

There are three types of audit.

Self-audit

Self-audit is carried out by individual members of the dental team or a group within the practice who are investigating their own care. The advantage is that team members can decide which topic they wish to investigate and hence the feeling of ownership is high. The main disadvantage is that because it is a private affair, collusion may occur and difficult questions may not be asked for fear of rocking the boat both professionally and personally. Hence important changes may be sacrificed for the sake of avoiding disruption.

Collaborative audit

In this process, colleagues from several practices get together to compare their audit findings in relation to a particular topic. Whereas self-audit addresses the questions, 'What do we do, why do we do it and do we actually do what we think we do?', collaborative audit adds the following question: 'Are we as competent as our peers?'

This consideration opens a new dimension and makes us take interest in how others achieve better results and how we might emulate them. Collaborative audit may appear more threatening and therefore of questionable benefit but colleagues from other practices may have a different mind-set and hence be able to offer approaches which we may not have considered. Comparisons need not be threatening because, as peer review has shown, dentists are usually keen to support and learn from each other. Very often, colleagues from other practices are quicker to find reasons to excuse our shortcomings than we are ourselves!

External audit

External audit differs from those described above because it is conducted by external assessors who bring with them a different perspective on our work. As yet, there is no formal system of external clinical audit within dentistry, although dental reference officers may provide feedback on clinical standards. An example of non-clinical external assessment is the IIP (Investors in People) award offered by the Learning Skills Council, which is finding favour with many dentists.

With external assessments, there is usually no scope for arguing with the criteria that have to be met, and only if we believe these criteria to be valid is the commitment worth considering.

☑ **Checkpoint 8.2**

External audit is a daunting prospect, but can offer advantages when compared to self-audit or collaborative audit. In your view, what do you think these might be?

☑ **Checkpoint 8.2 discussion**

Unlike self-audit or collaborative audit, external audits take a global view of how the practice functions. This means that not only are the separate components of healthcare examined, but also how well they fit together. There is a point to this, because unless team members are competent and the organisation fairly seamless, then the best quality care cannot be delivered. Such a wide-ranging audit is not within the scope of self-audit or collaborative audit and is therefore one advantage of submitting ourselves to external assessors.

External assessment is the most daunting prospect of those described, but the potential gains are also the greatest, resulting in improved self-esteem, better team-working and an enhanced reputation for the practice, justified because of the higher standards of care being delivered.

Think about external audits with which you are familiar – for example, charter marks such as Investors in People. If you are *not* considering undertaking an assessment of this sort, think about why this might be. We may consider the perceived workload to be the main barrier, but often the problem is to do with fear of being assessed and being found wanting. In reality, the intention of such assessments is to be formative and to help both individuals and teams to develop in line with common goals. This usually happens through the process of preparation rather than through the assessment itself. In addition, external assessments are usually associated with a support structure that ensures that the practice is not assessed until success (and the feel-good factor that goes with it) is guaranteed!

How do I conduct an audit?

Conducting an audit means undertaking a process which is best thought of as being ongoing, and is illustrated in Figure 8.1.

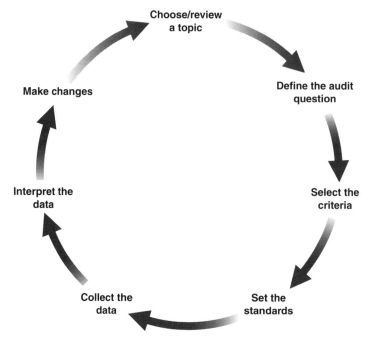

Figure 8.1 The audit cycle.

Choose a topic

The first thing to decide is what to audit. An appropriate subject should be one which:

- *Is important*: meaning that it is a clinical area which, if managed well, is likely to have significant benefits for the patients and the practice, or may have significant adverse consequences if managed poorly. Audit topics that are considered important by the team will have widespread commitment, which means that more help will be available to conduct the audit and more willingness will be shown to implement the recommendations. Audits that only reflect the personal interests of a small number will produce the opposite effects.

  When choosing a topic we might ask ourselves the following.

  - *In which areas of care do we have concerns regarding our performance?* Remember, though, that if harm has occurred or is likely, we should not fall into the trap of delaying action in order to await the outcomes of an audit. Initial measures can always be changed in the light of our audit recommendations.
  - *Which areas of care are being prioritised by the profession and society generally?*
  - *In which areas have significant advances recently been claimed?* For example, we might decide to test out the claims made for new dental materials by conducting an audit of crowns, looking for discoloration, subsequent decay or the number of remakes over a given period of time. Alternatively we could use a patient satisfaction questionnaire to determine if there was a problem with the retention of complete mandibular dentures. The new implant-retained dentures are said to be much better in this regard than conventional dentures and the audit results might encourage us to use this technique.

    The Faculty of General Dental Practitioners (UK) has produced a manual which general dental practitioners can use called *SAMS* (*The Self-assessment Manual and Standards*) and this provides a useful overview of the areas of clinical care that could be considered.

- *Has feasibility for improvement*: i.e. there are interventions which would improve on our current patient management, and that the expertise and resources to make use of the interventions are available.

- *Is measurable*: meaning that in relation to the topic being studied, there are elements that not only define performance, but can be measured reliably. Hence we might be able to audit our standard of root fillings by periodic post-operative radiographic analysis but we might find it almost impossible to audit the measures taken to reduce cross-infection. This is because of difficulties in measuring both the starting point and the changes that have occurred.

Define the audit question

Having decided on the general topic area we need to narrow this down to a specific audit question.

The purpose of doing this is that it allows us to set the criteria appropriately and specifically in line with the question we wish to answer. It also prevents us from asking a question that is so broad that it may prove unanswerable, leading to wasted time and a negative experience of audit. Of equal importance is the need to choose an audit question that we have the time, manpower and skill to investigate. Many audits leave a sour taste because they are too ambitious, and when conducting an audit for the first time, it is particularly important to start small enough to guarantee success and thereby develop faith in the process.

☑ **Checkpoint 8.3**

As an example of how to refine our task, let us suppose that we are interested in auditing our removable partial dentures. Our general topic area might be:

- *Are our removable partial dentures associated with significant deterioration of the oral tissues or surrounding muscles?*

Can you refine this further by producing specific audit questions?

> ☑ **Checkpoint 8.3 discussion**
>
> Here are some suggestions.
>
> We might decide to focus on *denture design*. It has been demonstrated that plaque accumulation at the vulnerable gingival margin is significantly reduced if the margin is not covered by part of the denture. In view of this, we might ask the following question:
>
> - *Is sufficient clearance of the gingival margin present?*
>
> Alternatively, we might choose to look at aspects of *continuing care* and ask:
>
> - *Are written instructions as well as verbal advice given on maintenance and aftercare?*
>
> Our topic area is principally concerned with the health of the oral tissues and we could audit this by considering the *plaque deposits* and asking:
>
> - *Is the level of plaque associated with the denture surfaces acceptably low?*
>
> Each of these questions will need to be associated with a reference point that can be measured, and we will consider the appropriate standards in a moment.

Selecting the criteria

The criteria are, quite simply, those items related to the audit question which can be measured or objectively assessed. Wherever possible, the criteria should be evidence-based or, at the very least, capable of being justified. For example, suppose that we wished to audit our removal of wisdom teeth. Suitable criteria that we could use might be those based on the guidelines produced by NICE (National Institute for Clinical Excellence).

Setting standards

When we define a criterion, it should be capable of having a standard attached, hence the importance of having an evidence-base from which to decide what the standard should be.

Very rarely is a standard of 100% appropriate in practice. We may initially wish to conduct an audit without setting a standard in order to establish a baseline. This is a practical approach that avoids us becoming disillusioned or overconfident if our initial standard was inappropriately high or low respectively. Usually, we try to set an *optimal* standard that is derived from a combination of:

- what the literature tells us represents good practice
- the implications of falling short of a gold standard
- what we know to be feasible given our resources and the characteristics of the communities we serve.

☑ **Checkpoint 8.4**

In Checkpoint 8.3, we considered removable partial dentures and produced three audit questions in relation to this topic. The questions were reasonable but, as no standard was attached, it would be impossible to undertake an audit. Here are the questions again. With respect to each of these audits, decide for yourself what the acceptable standards might be.

1 *Is sufficient clearance of the gingival margin present?*
2 *Are written instructions as well as verbal advice given on maintenance and aftercare?*
3 *Is the level of plaque associated with the denture surfaces acceptably low?*

☑ **Checkpoint 8.4 discussion**

1 *Is sufficient clearance of the gingival margin present?*

'Sufficient clearance' would have to be agreed by the clinicians involved. *SAMS* suggests a minimal acceptable standard (below which there is a potential for damage to the patient) of 3 mm clearance.

Our main concern is to make sure that every effort has been made to reach the desirable standard and we may therefore refine our audit question along the following lines.

- *With removable partial dentures, clearance of the gingival margin of at least 3 mm is either present or has been appropriately attempted in 60% of patients.*

Note that this audit is principally a measure of the clinical care provided by the dentist alone rather than the dental team.

2 *Are written instructions as well as verbal advice given on maintenance and aftercare?*

An appropriate standard could be 100%, but being able to achieve it will depend on having and implementing a practice protocol on continuing care as well as keeping records that such advice has been given.

This audit question looks more widely at the clinical care being provided by the team rather than the dentist alone.

3 *Is the level of plaque associated with the denture surfaces acceptably low?*

The problem here is to define 'acceptably low'. Unlike the previous two examples, the outcome of this audit will not only depend on the care offered by dentist and the team, but will also be influenced by patient compliance. In view of this, we may decide to set lower standards as our ability to improve the situation is limited. *SAMS* sets the level below which there is a potential for patient harm as the following.

Disclosing solution reveals deposits of plaque on < 20% of denture surfaces that contact teeth and gingival margins.

SAMS also defines the unacceptable level as 60% and, in view of this, we may decide to set a standard of between 20% and 60%, while obviously aiming for the highest standards that we can achieve.

Collecting the data

This can be collected from various sources such as reviewing the patients' notes, prospective data gathering, practice profiles issued by the Dental Practice Board and the use of questionnaires and interviews. When patient numbers are small e.g. fewer than 50, the aim could be to collect a complete data set. With larger numbers, a random sampling method such as examining every fifth record could be chosen. There is no rule regarding the absolute sample size, as this depends on the subject matter and how many in the practice population it relates to.

Interpreting the data

The object is to keep any analysis as simple as possible. Whereas we may present the data in tabular form or perhaps as a graph or histogram, formal statistical analysis should not be needed.

The purpose of interpretation is to answer the question 'Have we reached the performance standard or not?' If the standard has been reached, we should double-check that we didn't set the standard too low, and also ask ourselves what the concern was that prompted the initial inquiry. Might it have been that the criteria we chose were inappropriate and could not have addressed the initial question in the way we supposed?

If, as is usually the case, we have not attained the standard then the discussion should move on to consider the reasons why this might have been.

The way that the audit results are fed back needs careful thought. With clinical audit it is important that dentists can see how their performance compares with that of their colleagues, as this may be a significant motivator for change. To minimise the risk of embarrassment and loss of esteem, each dentist could be presented with a sheet of anonymised data showing comparisons between dentists. The person presenting the audit could maintain confidentiality by only allowing individuals to know which set of data refers to them.

Some dentists are less reserved and are willing to compare themselves more openly. Once dentists become more familiar with audit, this approach works better because it allows for a more fruitful discussion of why differences occur and how improvements can be made.

Presenting the data

The object of presenting the data is to make the results of the audit clear and to facilitate interpretation and discussion. For these reasons, it is best not to obscure the main messages by presenting too much information and care should be taken to display the data honestly and clearly. The audit example at the end of this chapter shows how this can be done with simple tables, a histogram and straightforward interpretation.

Making changes

Once we have swallowed our pride and recognised that there is room for improvement we should turn our attention to how this might be achieved. It may be the case that in order to reach the audit standard, improvement is only required of isolated individuals, in which case the changes needed can be addressed by these individuals through their PDPs. More often, however, the improvements required are more generalised, involving several people and affecting the management of clinical care as well as its content.

In these situations, we must first decide whether the changes needed to achieve the improvement are worth the effort expended. We only have limited resources (meaning time, finances and energy) and we cannot make all the improvements that are possible. Therefore there should be consensus when the priorities for the practice are chosen. The changes proposed must be feasible and they must also be fair to all concerned. Hence it might be inappropriate for a partner who seldom undertakes periodontal work to insist that those who do should routinely use full-pocket charting.

Review of the topic

Having decided on the changes we wish to implement, we set new standards which will be more realistic and probably higher than the first time round, and conduct a further audit. This process, which allows us to check whether agreed changes are being implemented, is called completing the audit cycle or 'closing the loop'.

Continuous monitoring

When audits are repeated, they are done periodically, usually after a set period of time. Nowadays, with the increasing sophistication of practice computers, there are electronic systems which allow for continuous monitoring of various parameters either pre-programmed in the software or set by the practice.

This procedure is not widespread but continuous monitoring could not only allow important areas of care to be kept under surveillance, such as the longevity of restorations in relation to the material used, but also allow trends to be recognised. When necessary, corrective action could be taken before a problem develops. Continuous monitoring could help us to look at our individual performance, the management of individual patients and also the healthcare delivered to larger groups.

When conducting an audit in a computerised practice, it is always worth considering whether the audit could be done electronically, either on the first occasion or when closing the loop. If we have this in mind, we can gradually build up the database that allows future audits to be performed more easily and, possibly, automatically.

An example of dental audit

Audit title

'Do patients understand their treatment charges?'

Why was this audit chosen?

1 We occasionally have problems that result from patients questioning their treatment charges. One significant event in which the patient refused to pay prompted us to investigate our procedures.

2 It is also a Terms of Service requirement for dentists to inform patients appropriately and to issue form FP17DC if:

- part of the treatment is to be provided privately
- prolonged periodontal treatment is involved
- three or more fillings are to be provided
- endodontics is involved
- a veneer, inlay or bridge is to be provided
- surgical treatment is to be provided (other than extractions)
- extraction of two or more teeth is planned or if any difficult extractions are needed

- a denture is to be provided
- orthodontic treatment is required
- if the patient requests one.

This form sets out what treatment under the NHS contract is needed, what the patient charges are and, if any treatment is also being carried out privately, what this is and what the private charges are.

It also details what patients are required to do, such as to pay the dentist the NHS charges due and to attend for appointments.

Aims

The aims of the audit were to see to what degree with respect to each of the dentists in the practice:

- form FP17DC was appropriately issued
- patients understood what they were paying for.

Standards

Standard 1

Ninety per cent of patients in the study group should receive form FP17DC at the outset of their treatment.

Standard 2

Ninety per cent of patients should understand the treatment estimate given to them at the outset of their treatment.

Methods

In this audit, the source material and references included:

- NHS (General Dental Services) Regulations 1992
- form FP17DC
- the manual *SAMS*
- patient record cards, FP25a.

At our practice, there are three dentists with NHS contract numbers and two part-time receptionists.

During the audit, data was collected prospectively on 100 patients for each dentist, this number being sufficient to provide a representative sample of our practice population. These were the first 100 patients identified by each practitioner for whom they felt form FP17DC would be needed according to the criteria listed above.

The dentists made a record of the identity of these patients (the study group) and the type of treatment (private, NHS or mixed) but did not alert the receptionist to these facts until the end of the study.

The patient was then sent to the receptionist who made a decision as to whether form FP17DC was required. She based this decision upon information provided by the dentist either verbally or via the patient record card.

Whenever form FP17DC was issued, the receptionist asked the patient whether he understood the treatment that was proposed and the financial implications.

Data relating to this was collected on a specially designed form completed by the receptionist and cross-referenced at the end of the audit with the details of the study group held by the dentists.

Results

Table 8.1

Dentist	A	B	C	Average
NHS treatments	88	90	100	93
Private	9	8	0	5
Mixed NHS/private	3	2	0	2
Total	100	100	100	100

Table 8.2

Dentist	A	B	C	Average
FP17DC issued	89	57	84	77
Patient understands the treatment charges	88	54	64	69

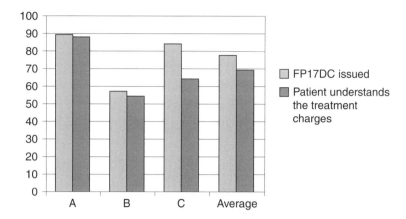

Figure 8.2 Audit of treatment charges.

Discussion

- Complete data was available on all the subjects in this audit, which suggests good data collection, particularly by the receptionists.
- Table 8.1 indicates the treatment types. The majority of patients (93%) included in the audit received NHS treatment, which is a fair representation of our work pattern. One dentist had seen no private patients.
- Table 8.2 shows how well we performed according to our audit standards. The figures in the 'average' column indicate that we fell short as a practice of our standard of 90% with respect to appropriately issuing form FP17DC (77%) and ensuring that patients understand the estimate (69%).
- This is disappointing overall, but obscures the variation between individual dentists in the practice. We discussed the interpretation of these results as a dental team and came to the following conclusions.

Dentist A

This dentist seemed to inform the reception staff very well and was not far short of the first audit standard. He also had very high scores for patient understanding and almost all the patients who received a form understood its implications. Dentist A said that he routinely counselled patients and confirmed that they were happy with the treatment proposed and its cost implications. However, probably as a result of this, he said that he had problems with keeping to time and often ran late.

Dentist B

This dentist performed relatively poorly and fell well short of both standards. The receptionists reported that little verbal communication occurred and that the patient record cards were either not legible or not complete. The dentist reported that he used an abbreviation in the cards that was meant to alert receptionists to fill in form FP17DC. Unfortunately, the receptionists were not aware of this system as it was not in routine use with the other dentists in the practice.

In this audit, the second audit criterion is dependent upon the first. The fewer patients that receive a treatment estimate form, the fewer are questioned about their understanding of it. With this in mind, although dentist B scored poorly for the first criterion, his communication with patients was very good and nearly all his patients said that they understood the treatment. As with dentist A, dentist B said that he routinely advised patients about the proposed treatment.

Dentist C

This dentist did well with keeping receptionists informed and was noted by them to have very clear and readable records. Unfortunately, a relatively high percentage of his patients who were questioned stated that they did not understand the treatment that they were recommended to have. Interestingly, the significant event that prompted this audit involved a patient of this dentist. This dentist is new to the practice and he said that he had assumed the receptionists gave some information on treatment costs to patients.

NHS v private treatment

We undertook a separate analysis (not shown) comparing our performance of patients who had NHS treatments alone versus private treatment alone. We found that for 16 out of 17 of the private patients in this audit, both standards were fully achieved.

Action plan

This audit was effectively an assessment of communication between team members and between dentists and patients. As a team, we felt that everyone had demonstrated aspects of good practice that were worthy of commendation. We also recognised that, to improve matters, we would need to work more co-operatively and share our ideas and expectations. Following a team meeting, we decided to do the following.

- Agree on *one* system to alert receptionists that form FP17DC needed completion.
- Educate receptionists so that they can independently check whether the criteria for FP17DC have been met.
- Ensure that our records are legible.
- Produce a practice leaflet that would give further information on treatment charges.
- Routinely check that patients have understood the treatment charges.
- Undertake a re-audit six months after implementing these changes.
- Discuss the results at a future team meeting.

Who can help me?

From 24 May 2001, as part of clinical governance in general dental practice, it became a Terms of Service requirement for all general dental practitioners on a health authority list in England, including assistants and vocational dental practitioners, to carry out 15 hours of audit or peer review in a rolling three-year programme.

All practitioners are funded for this activity under the government-funded Clinical Audit and Peer Review Scheme. Full details are available on the NCCPED website, www.nccped.co.uk, and further information is also available on the BDA site, bda-dentistry.org.uk.

The scheme is overseen centrally by a Central Assessment Panel (CAP) and locally by Local Assessment Panels (LAPs).

The CAP has set up a network of audit facilitators around the country and practitioners wanting help and advice in carrying out an audit in their practice can access these facilitators through their local LAP. A number of dentists have received appropriate training to undertake the role of Clinical Audit Facilitator. Their role is not to audit a practice but to be available to provide help, advice and support for dentists who wish to undertake audit.

Although there are differences in the way that they operate, similar schemes are running in Wales, Scotland and Northern Ireland.

Summary

Unlike significant events, which demand our attention, audit is less dramatic in that it does not proclaim its importance and brings its rewards over a longer timescale. It is nevertheless a powerful method by which to plan and monitor improvements in care and so valuable is it considered to be that audit activity is likely to form part of the requirement for revalidation. Most dentists are perpetually interested in their work and in the standards which their practices achieve, and audit is a natural extension of this interest. When audit is unsuccessful, it is usually because the audit question was too big, but provided the question is clearly focused and the audit cycle is followed, the experience of audit should be a positive and useful one.

When engaging in audit for the first time, dentists are often surprised as to how simple it is, but as we have seen throughout this book, nearly all the techniques we use to further our education are straightforward and within everyone's grasp.

Further information

- The rules and procedures regarding clinical audit and peer review are clearly laid out on the BDA website: http://www.bda-dentistry.org.uk/.

- The details of the Department of Health Clinical Audit and Peer Review Scheme in the GDS in England in April 2001 are available in a handbook from: http://www.doh.gov.uk/pdfs/moddent.pdf.

- An example of publication standard, *A Clinical Audit into the Success Rate of Inferior Alveolar Nerve Block Analgesia in General Dental Practice*, by A Keetley and DR Moles, can be seen at: http://www.rcseng.ac.uk/dental/fgdp/pdc/pdf/report_8_4.pdf.

- Baker R, Hearnshaw H and Robertson N (eds) (1999) *Implementing Change with Clinical Audit.* John Wiley & Sons, Chichester.

  This book looks particularly at the barriers to change and how they might be overcome. The examples are from general medical practice although the principles are relevant to dental care.

9 Appraisal: moving beyond the PDP

Key points

■ Appraisal is a process whereby colleagues meet on a regular basis to review their performance and plan next year's PDP.

■ Appraisals are usually annual, and can be conducted in an individual or a group setting.

■ The process involves recognising and applauding achievements.

- The appraisee can be appraised as an individual, a dentist and as a team member.
- The appraisal is based on evaluations conducted by the appraisee, including evaluation of the last year's PDP.
- Later on, asking colleagues to make evaluations of our performance can greatly increase its value.
- Evaluations are used in a structured appraisal meeting to highlight strengths and weaknesses that are then discussed with the appraiser.
- Appraisers should be colleagues who have both sufficient insight and the respect of the appraisee. They need not be dentists.
- Appraisers need to be skilled in listening and providing feedback.
- The appraisal meeting results in specific objectives being produced for next year's PDP, a summary of the meeting being written and a future appraisal date being agreed.
- Particularly at the outset, appraisals should be kept very simple, with the emphasis on support rather than criticism – our first experience of appraisal should not also be our last!

Why bother?

As a concept, appraisal is not new to dentists. We may already have come across staff appraisals in which, usually on an annual basis, time is put aside for the employee to discuss with a more senior manager or employer his progress during the year. The opportunity is taken to recognise and applaud achievement (the 'praise' in the word 'appraisal'), to give constructive feedback and to encourage the employee to develop further.

Despite providing the opportunity to take stock of our lives and attempt to gain some control over them, most dentists don't flock to the idea of appraisal, and the reasons are understandable. First, the process seems alien – dirty linen was never intended to be washed in public and, anyway, isn't it all a bit too much like navel gazing? Second, who among us is fit to sit in judgement on our peers? Third, even if we could find someone to do the appraising, isn't there the danger that criticism (however tentatively voiced) might seriously undermine the appraisee? These fears are not unfounded, but it *can* be said that provided the process is kept simple and the appraiser observes certain straightforward rules, appraisal can do much to help dentists develop as people and as professionals.

In the medical community, where NHS appraisal of general medical practitioners and hospital consultants became compulsory in 2002, the process has been led by the profession and has kept its focus on educational development. It has not been allowed to become 'performance review' in which the performance of professionals is measured against externally imposed criteria, but has been based around the professional development of the individual. As a result, appraisal for doctors is based on the PDP with which you are now familiar. At the end of this chapter, we will look at this linkage in more detail and discover how appraisal is the natural progression from the PDP.

For doctors, it has also been established that the satisfactory completion of five annual appraisals, each of which involves the discussion of the PDP, should provide enough evidence for revalidation. Thus good-quality CPD should be sufficient to demonstrate fitness to practise.

Summary points

Appraisal is worth doing because it helps us to:

- review our performance over the past year using our completed PDP
- receive constructive criticism and advice
- improve relationships with those with whom we work
- increase our job satisfaction and prevent burnout
- plan our development for the coming year and write our next PDP.

Introductory exercise

In this chapter, we will see how appraisal can help our personal and professional development. We will consider how appraisals can be performed and look at the documentation that might be used. However, before going any further, we should recognise that, for dentists, appraisal may seem to be a threatening process, more concerned with assessment and negative criticism than acknowledgement of success and constructive planning for the future. In fact, it is the latter which characterises appraisal, and to demonstrate this for ourselves, it is worth undertaking the following exercise.

Arrange with a colleague to conduct a mutual appraisal exercise. No homework is required – just find a comfortable place to sit where you will be uninterrupted for one hour and go through the following process. Taking it in turns, one colleague will do the talking while the other asks the questions listed below, listening attentively and only offering comments when invited to do so. The questioner can use a proforma to record his impressions *see* Appendix 1).

First person: think about yourself as a clinician/manager/team member and answer the following questions (20 minutes).

- In your professional life, what do you consider that you are doing well?
- During the past 12 months, what would you consider to have been your major achievement at work?
- What part of your job do you find most difficult?
- During the past 12 months, what would you consider to have been your major disappointment?
- What would you need in order to improve your effectiveness?

Second person: summarise the key points made, checking with the first person that the summary is accurate (5 minutes).

Reverse roles, taking a further 25 minutes.

Jointly discuss impressions of the process (10 minutes). These can be noted on the proforma if desired.

- How did it feel?
- What were your prior concerns about the process – were they justified?
- Are you interested in developing the process further?

Hopefully, some of your fears will have been allayed and you will have experienced the 'buzz' that many clinicians do when given an opportunity to talk about their concerns and aspirations with a respected peer who has put time aside for the purpose. In the following discussion, we will use this experience and show how appraisal builds on it in three ways:

- by getting us to do some preparatory work designed to identify our strengths and weaknesses
- by encouraging the appraiser to be more challenging
- by devoting more time to setting future objectives and planning how these might be met.

What is the process of appraisal?

Before examining this in more detail, it is useful at this point to have an overview of the process from the appraisee's perspective.

Stage	Comments
1 Choose an appraiser	Either an individual or group
2 Set a date for the appraisal	Usually on an annual basis
3 Decide which areas are to be evaluated	This may concern our performance as an individual/dentist/team member
4 Conduct the evaluations	This will always include self-evaluation and may include feedback from others
5 Review the evaluations	Any feedback forms will also be reviewed by the appraiser
6 Attend the appraisal meeting	This will follow a pre-defined format
7 Plan the future objectives	These are principally owned by the appraisee
8 Start again!	

Let us now consider the main stages.

Who can conduct an appraisal?

Appraisals can be conducted either as individual interviews or as group activities, and there are advantages and disadvantages to both. The dentist has the choice of who appraises him. Key points are that whoever is involved in appraising must understand and respect the rules of giving feedback (discussed below), and whichever approach is chosen, there needs to be protected time, sufficient time and an agreed process.

For most people, despite the labour-intensive approach of individual interviews, this method may be preferred, at least at the outset. This is because the environment is less threatening, which is an important consideration when we are new to the process. The appraiser must be respected and credible in the eyes of the appraisee, but need not be another dentist. Indeed, practice managers could be used as appraisers particularly when the review does not require specialist clinical knowledge, as they have much knowledge of the working of the team and a broader perspective on the practice and partnership. Whoever we choose, it can be better to select someone whose outlook is not identical to our own. This helps to prevent appraisal being too cosy, because without some degree of challenge we are unlikely to make progress.

For dentists who are single-handed or from small practices, either non-dental staff (e.g. the practice nurse or manager) or a colleague from another practice could act as appraiser, perhaps on a reciprocal basis.

The advantages of the individual interview are that, as well as feeling safe, it has greater confidentiality and may allow more time for personal attention than in a group setting. However, because of the lack of other participants, feedback may be less broad-based and representative. Because of the intimate nature of individual encounters, the appraiser might also find criticism more difficult to voice than in a group.

For those who conduct appraisals in a group, the time allowed for each individual may only be 20 minutes. On the other hand, group appraisal is more time-efficient and can improve team-working because everyone receives some criticism and some praise, and the needs of the *team* can be taken into account when the future plans of the *individual* are made. These benefits are attractive, but facilitating such a meeting requires a fair degree of skill! Whichever form of appraisal is chosen, the process is confidential and is not reported to outsiders such as peer-review groups unless all those involved wish it to happen.

What areas could be covered in an appraisal?

We may choose to be appraised on areas such as:

- *clinical care*: looking at the care of individuals, e.g. through case analysis and significant event analysis
- *communication skills*: in which we look at both verbal and written communication with patients and team members, perhaps through the use of questionnaires
- *record keeping*: in which we check that we record our patient contacts and keep notes that are comprehensive and legible
- *practice roles and responsibilities*: whereby we compare our achievements against the tasks for which we are responsible
- *team-working*: in which we assess our commitment to team-working through attendance at team meetings, awareness of skills within the team, appropriate delegation, the completion of appointed tasks and so on
- *continuing professional development*: perhaps by reviewing our PDP or looking at our role in the development of the practice
- *career progression*: looking at our medium- and long-term personal goals.

How do we decide which areas to choose?

Clearly, not all these areas can be covered in one appraisal (unless we are prepared to spend a weekend over it!). In deciding which areas to review, we may wish to take some of the following factors into account.

Does the appraisal have a specific purpose?

For some dentists, appraisal may be restricted to a particular area – for example, CPD, in which case the goals of reviewing learning objectives and checking for evidence of learning are fairly straightforward. For others, appraisal may be an opportunity to look more generally at our work, perhaps by selecting two or three areas from those listed above. Sometimes individuals will decide with their appraisers which aspects of their work they wish to discuss. Alternatively, particularly where appraisal is a practice commitment, the group may decide on the areas in which they wish the members to be appraised.

Do we review our work in any other settings?

Our choice of appraisal areas will partly depend on the availability of other review/evaluation meetings during the year. Hence if we have specific meetings to share the results of audit and learn from them, we may choose to leave this element out of our appraisal meeting.

Are there any areas of our work that are best discussed in private?

Appraisals are a valuable opportunity for discussing personal goals or evaluations that may be difficult to consider in other settings because of their sensitive nature. Such evaluations may include feedback on our professionalism from staff and colleagues. This opportunity applies particularly to appraisals that are conducted as individual interviews.

NHS appraisals for general medical practitioners require doctors to complete a lengthy (but helpful) form that includes many of the areas of consideration listed above. This can be viewed at the website: www.appraisaluk.info and is relevant to dentists as well as to doctors.

Why are evaluations needed for appraisal?

If the objective of being appraised is to help us to improve, then as a starting point we need to have an idea of our strengths and weaknesses. Having decided on the scope of our appraisal, some form of evaluation is required and two choices are immediately available to us. The first is self-evaluation, which is non-threatening, relatively easy to conduct and can take various forms such as:

- answering a subjective questionnaire (*see* Appendix 2 and Appendix 3)
- reviewing our individual case management or our significant events
- analysing the results of audit.

The second is to involve others in the evaluation process. They may do so by analysing the work of the practice, perhaps by conducting audit, or may provide feedback on our performance by completing questionnaires. When dentists are compared with colleagues on the basis of data, protests about its use are relatively muted as data is objective. Feedback, however, is a different proposition as it could be subjective, personal and potentially damaging. These may seem to be good reasons to avoid its use, but that would be a pity because feedback adds a much broader and potentially useful dimension to evaluation.

Summary points

The feedback process has the ability to:

- give us insights regarding our performance that cannot be gained by self-reflection
- encourage contributors to be constructive
- increase respect for our professionalism
- improve team-working by demonstrating that we care about the views of our colleagues and patients
- increase the support that we receive from our colleagues in everyday life, and in meeting the objectives identified through appraisal.

Unlike analysing data, the feedback forms that others complete can tell us much about those aspects of professional life that are difficult to measure, such as our understanding of roles, ability to follow protocols, our motivation, enthusiasm, readiness to accept change and so on.

We will look at how to conduct appraisal that incorporates both self-evaluation *and* the feedback of others, but it is recommended that you start with self-evaluation alone and add feedback later, when the process of appraisal is more familiar to you.

The fact that evaluation plays a role means that appraisal is quite different from pure mentoring (with which it is sometimes confused) which, despite having similar aims of support and development, is devoid of an evaluation function. However, the human skills that good mentors must have, particularly communication skills such as active listening, are also important to good appraisers, as we will see later.

How do we conduct the evaluations?

Self-evaluation

An important part of self-evaluation is to complete a proforma (*see* Appendix 2) that looks in general terms at our performance as individuals, dentists and team members.

Other evaluations will require varying amounts of work depending on the areas chosen for appraisal. Hence reviewing our strengths and weaknesses in clinical practice may lead us to audit our work or complete a rating scale in which we rate our confidence at dealing with a range of conditions important in general dental practice. Rating scales can also be used to assess our confidence with other aspects of professional life such as communication, organisation, professional values and personal and professional growth.

Two examples of useful rating scales known as the 'self-evaluation questionnaires' or SEQs are shown in Appendix 3 and cover clinical areas as well as management and administration.

The conclusions that we draw from these evaluations and take with us to the appraisal meeting should be fairly general, because appraisal is not intended to be a forum in which minutiae (such as the results of a clinical audit) are discussed, but rather an opportunity to overview our work.

Feedback from others

This may involve asking the perspective of employees, attached staff and patients. For those dentists who have wider responsibilities it may also mean asking the views of other peers, employers and those to whom we provide a service. This wide-ranging input is sometimes referred to as '360° feedback', but it is not mandatory to commit ourselves to this process. As a beginning, it is quite acceptable to narrow our focus and to ask a selected group – some feedback is a great deal better than none at all.

Depending on the size of the organisation, we may wish to invite everyone within our chosen group(s) to contribute, or if the group is large we may ask a select few. At least three people would be required to ensure anonymity and thereby encourage contribution. It is worth taking advice from the group regarding who would be suitable contributors, with the aims of obtaining a range of opinions and choosing people who are more likely to be objective in their outlook. Our contributors need to be representative of the whole, so for example if we were to seek the views of our employees, we would want to hear from dental nurses and receptionists, the practice manager, dental hygienist, etc.

What, then, would we ask them and what sort of responses might we get? This depends on the area of inquiry, so for example if we were to ask our dental colleagues about our record keeping they might conduct a brief audit and provide us with factual feedback. Alternatively, our colleagues might be asked a question such as how we seem to cope with stress, to which the answer would be a matter of subjective opinion. Remembering that some of the most important questions do not have factual answers, we should try not to dismiss subjectivity – after all, the impressions that others have of us are as close to 'reality' as our own perceptions. Differences between the views of others and our own perceptions may highlight facets of our performance worthy of further consideration.

Because improvement is the objective of appraisal, and improvement means change, when formulating the questions we must avoid asking about areas of our performance or behaviour where change is not possible. For example, our personalities are fixed (whatever we may hope) although our punctuality might be improved on.

To improve the value of feedback, it is important that the contributions are anonymous. Although there is a concern that the disgruntled might use this as an opportunity to 'have a go', in reality most people seek to be helpful. Unwarranted flattery is equally unhelpful, although most dentists would probably not see this as being of particular concern!

The questions that are asked can be developed from our own perspective, but it is useful to involve the group that we are going to question. They can check that the questions are appropriate and answerable, and can also advise as to whether any important areas of inquiry have been omitted. Alternatively, we may wish to allow our colleagues to devise a questionnaire of their own. Once the questionnaires have been distributed, *we* should also complete them so as to make comparisons in the next stage.

An example of a comprehensive 360° feedback form is shown in Appendix 6. This can be used as it stands or edited to a more manageable size to concentrate on particular areas.

How do we review the feedback?

When the feedback evaluations are completed, they should be returned to the appraisee (the person being appraised) and a copy sent to the appraiser. Both will have an opportunity to evaluate the responses and pick out any common themes, average out the scores given on rating scales and highlight any important points that might have been made. In addition, we will be able to compare these evaluations with our self-evaluation and decide how much truth we think there is, good and bad, in what people have said about us. Alternatively, the feedback forms can be analysed by the appraisee and this evaluation sent to the appraiser.

From this and from our other self-evaluations, including the evaluation of last year's PDP, we are now in a position to decide what we wish to discuss in the appraisal meeting, bearing in mind that it is important to choose problem areas where change is possible. If we do not, there is a danger that the meeting will be inconclusive and we will feel demoralised, having done little more than identify difficulties that we are powerless to act on.

Summary points

Reviewing the evaluations allows us to:

- see ourselves as others see us
- evaluate discrepancies and decide whether comments are justified
- look at our relationships across the team – do we seem to have problems with a particular group?
- identify our learning needs in preparation for writing next year's PDP.

How do we prepare ourselves for the appraisal?

Having conducted and reviewed the evaluations, it is important to go into the appraisal meeting with an appropriate attitude.

The evaluation exercise will have uncovered much that is good and some that could be better, and it is important to remember both elements and to avoid being too self-critical. Dentists rarely receive praise from their colleagues and appraisal is one mechanism of ensuring that good work is recognised and applauded by someone whose opinion matters to the appraisee. Although rather un-British it is just as important for dentists to recognise their *own* worth. As well as allowing for criticism, appraisal encourages us to comment on those things we feel we do well, and to pat ourselves on the back for them. For some, accepting praise may be more uncomfortable than accepting criticism, but it is just as important a part of being honest with ourselves.

At the appraisal meeting, its positive purpose, which is to plan our future development through the PDP, should be borne in mind as this encourages us to be constructive rather than defensive, to listen to the observations of our colleagues and to make suggestions of our own.

How should the appraisal meeting be conducted?

There are three elements to this that we will discuss separately – the ground rules, the structure of the meeting and the skills required by the appraiser.

Ground rules

Find a comfortable place to sit, and make sure that enough uninterrupted time is allocated for the task. The meeting should follow a planned format of which all parties are aware and the rules regarding record keeping and confidentiality should be made explicit.

Structure of the meeting

A suggested structure which could be used for both individual interviews and group meetings is shown in Appendix 4, in which the comments made regarding the appraiser also apply to team members who are providing feedback in group appraisals. At each stage, the appraisee should speak first.

For individual interviews, the process might take up to two hours, but for group interviews the time that each dentist has is usually much shorter, perhaps 20 minutes. The appraiser should keep brief notes so that a short written summary can be prepared after the meeting and a form such as that in Appendix 5 can serve both purposes.

Appraiser skills

Appraisers need to use many of the same skills required for patient-centred consulting. They should establish rapport, let the appraisee speak without undue interruption, maintain eye contact and avoid being patronising. In addition to this, the fact that appraisal involves criticism – constructive criticism, but criticism nevertheless – can't be avoided. To prevent the harmful effects of this, the appraiser should bear in mind the following points.

- Criticism should not be a surprise – the ground rules should make it clear that this is part of the process.
- Criticism should only come after the initial positive evaluation of the appraisee.
- The appraisee should be encouraged to be self-critical and make his own suggestions for improvement.
- Wherever possible, criticism should be based on facts, using specific examples from the feedback received and from other evaluations.
- The manner in which criticism is given, i.e. its language and tone, is important.
- The value of an appraiser to an appraisee is enhanced if appropriate criticism is not avoided.

When giving feedback, appraisers should use clear language, avoid prejudice or bias and discuss areas that are amenable to change. Improvements between current and previous performance should be recognised and applauded and any objectives agreed upon should be attainable.

Those who act as appraisers can improve their skills by getting some feedback after the appraisal meeting. This feedback can cover the nature of the interaction such as the quality of listening, the aids or hindrances to communication and the way in which criticism was offered.

What happens afterwards?

After the meeting, the appraiser should use his notes to prepare a short summary (*see* Appendix 5) whose contents can be agreed with the appraisee. A copy can then be kept by both. It is usually intended that the objectives that have been agreed be written in the PDP and achieved in time for the next appraisal meeting.

Summary points

The outcomes of appraisal are:

* recognition of good practice and the goals that we have achieved
* identification of areas in which improvement is needed
* setting specific objectives that we can include in our PDPs
* support from our colleagues in achieving these objectives.

Appraisal and the PDP

At the start of the chapter, it was suggested that appraisal is the natural progression beyond the PDP. This assertion is partly based on evidence from the medical community, where there is an explicit tie-in between the two processes, as shown in Figure 9.1, but also from the experience of dentists. The Hillsborough group in Sheffield (not all of whom are Sheffield Wednesday supporters!) are a peer-review group who have conducted mutual appraisal not because it was being recommended but because they recognised a need to discuss the professional and personal factors that influence their career development. As with doctors, for whom appraisal is compulsory, their experience has been that appraisal allows a wider and more informed discussion of personal needs from which a more useful PDP can be developed. In addition, and most importantly, appraisal provides a great sense of support from the professional community and can improve job satisfaction.

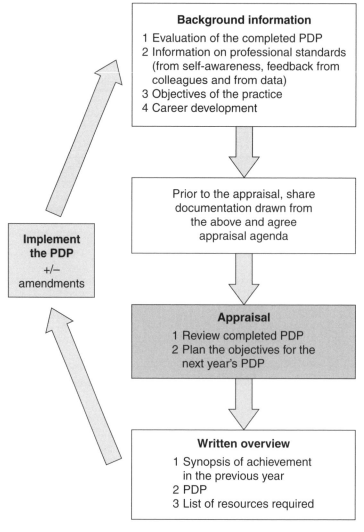

Figure 9.1 Appraisal and the link with the PDP.

Looking at Figure 9.1, we can see how the continuous process of professional development links with annual appraisal. We can use a range of sources to provide the background information needed for appraisal. These include reflection on the outcomes of the previous year's PDP (the 'completed PDP'), an evaluation of personal performance and a consideration of where we wish to be. The latter is determined with reference to personal developmental aspirations, and also through consideration of where and how the practice needs to develop.

By reflecting on this information and sharing some or all of it with our appraiser, we can decide which areas we particularly wish to discuss in the appraisal meeting. The meeting itself may be broad-ranging, but has clear objectives that help to keep us on track. It ends with identification and agreement of the learning needs and associated objectives for next year's PDP as well as the resources it may require.

A mutually agreed record of the appraisal meeting along with the new PDP set us on course for our CPD for the coming year. During the year we implement the plan, develop new abilities and collect evidence of our learning. Finally, we end with an evaluation of the year's activities and use this to inform the next appraisal.

Summary

So, there we have it – an overview of appraisal demonstrating the potential benefits to dentists and their colleagues. To keep the process concise, useful and enjoyable, follow these steps:

- Complete the introductory exercise.
- Discuss with your colleagues which areas you would like to appraise.
- Keep your initial evaluations simple.
- Have a go at appraisal using the suggested structure for the meeting and then base your PDP on the outcome of the appraisal meeting.

Later, as we become more confident, we can think about requesting feedback about our performance from the people we work with and about improving our skills as appraisers. Finally, remember that, far from being a destructive process, praise from those who have our permission to be critical does much to boost our self-esteem. We could even say that appraisal is good for our health!

Further information

Haman H, Irvine S and Jelley D (2001) *The Peer Appraisal Handbook for General Practitioners.* Radcliffe Medical Press, Oxford.

A useful text on the process of appraisal which gives more detail on the methods of collecting evidence and conducting a successful appraisal interview.

Appendix 1
Appraisal: introductory exercise

Think about yourself as a clinician/manager/ team member and answer the following.

Name:

Question	Notes
In your professional life, what do you consider that you are doing well?	*Clinician* *Manager* *Team member*
During the past 12 months, what would you consider to have been your major achievement at work?	
What part of your job do you find most difficult?	
During the past 12 months, what would you consider to have been your major disappointment?	
What would you need in order to improve your effectiveness?	*Clinician* *Manager* *Team member*

Your impressions of appraisal
How did it feel?
What were your prior concerns about the process – were they justified?
Are you interested in developing the process further?

Appendix 2 Dentist's self-evaluation

This form should be completed prior to the appraisal meeting.

As a dentist

What do you consider that you are doing well?

How do you know?

What part of your job do you find most difficult?

What skills would you need to improve your effectiveness?

As a member of the healthcare team

What are your strengths in terms of team-working?

What are your weaknesses?

What are the barriers to your improvement?

As an individual

How might you cope better with stress?

How might you manage your time better?

What obstacles are preventing you from doing a better job?

During the past 12 months, what would you consider to have been your major achievement?

During the past 12 months, what would you consider to have been your major disappointment?

During the next 12 months, what are your personal, educational and practice goals?

How do you plan to achieve these goals?

What resources might you require?

Appendix 3
Self-evaluation
questionnaires (SEQs)

Identifying learning needs: clinical

Name:

Please read the questions below and select the option that most accurately reflects how you feel.

Using the following 'blob' system, please fill in the 'knowledge' and 'ability' boxes below.

-   •   I don't feel I know a lot/I am not confident I achieve this.
-   ••   I feel my knowledge is adequate/I am reasonable at achieving this.
- ••• I feel my knowledge is (very) good/I am good at achieving this.

Then put a ✓ against your two most pressing priorities.

	Knowledge	Ability	Priority?
Taking a medical history	☐	☐	☐
Full mouth examination	☐	☐	☐
Periodontal examination	☐	☐	☐
Periodontal monitoring	☐	☐	☐
Oral cancer check	☐	☐	☐
Use of local anaesthetic	☐	☐	☐
Reviewing radiographs	☐	☐	☐
Treatment planning	☐	☐	☐
Oral hygiene instruction	☐	☐	☐
Patient motivation	☐	☐	☐
Scaling and maintenance	☐	☐	☐
Extractions	☐	☐	☐
Root planing	☐	☐	☐
Cavity preparation	☐	☐	☐
Placement of amalgam restorations	☐	☐	☐
Placement of anterior restorations	☐	☐	☐
Crown preparation	☐	☐	☐
Bridge preparation	☐	☐	☐
Endodontic treatment	☐	☐	☐
Taking impressions for advanced work	☐	☐	☐
Occlusal adjustment	☐	☐	☐
Construction of complete dentures	☐	☐	☐
Construction of partial dentures (acrylic)	☐	☐	☐
Construction of partial dentures (metal)	☐	☐	☐
Orthodontic diagnosis and evaluation	☐	☐	☐
Oral pathology	☐	☐	☐
Oral surgery	☐	☐	☐
Treating children	☐	☐	☐
Implants	☐	☐	☐
First-aid procedures	☐	☐	☐
Communication skills	☐	☐	☐
Cross-infection control procedures	☐	☐	☐
Keeping up to date with new techniques	☐	☐	☐

Identifying learning needs: management and administration

Name:

Please read the questions below and select the option that most accurately reflects how you feel.

Using the following 'blob' system, please fill in the 'knowledge' and 'ability' boxes below.

- •   I don't feel I know a lot/I am not confident I achieve this.
- ••   I feel my knowledge is adequate/I am reasonable at achieving this.
- ••• I feel my knowledge is (very) good/I am good at achieving this.

Then put a ✓ against your two most pressing priorities in each section.

	Knowledge	Ability	Priority?
Management			
Prepare a ten-year strategic plan	☐	☐	☐
Prepare a two-year strategic plan	☐	☐	☐
Carry out a SWOT analysis	☐	☐	☐
Set SMART objectives	☐	☐	☐
Delegate to staff	☐	☐	☐
Monitor and evaluate individual performance	☐	☐	☐
Organise and prioritise own workload	☐	☐	☐
Time management	☐	☐	☐
Create and maintain effective relationships with staff	☐	☐	☐
Create and maintain effective relationships with patients	☐	☐	☐
Manage stress	☐	☐	☐
Manage customer care	☐	☐	☐
Solve problems	☐	☐	☐
Run effective practice meetings	☐	☐	☐
Plan on a day-to-day basis	☐	☐	☐
Awareness of health and safety issues	☐	☐	☐
Maintain quality of service	☐	☐	☐

	Knowledge	Ability	Priority?
Administration			
Making an appointment for a patient	☐	☐	☐
Setting up office management systems	☐	☐	☐
Using the filing system	☐	☐	☐
Organising the recall system	☐	☐	☐
Typing a business letter	☐	☐	☐
Using a Dictaphone	☐	☐	☐
Writing a referral letter	☐	☐	☐
Keyboard skills on computer	☐	☐	☐
Knowledge and use of word processing	☐	☐	☐
Knowledge and use of spreadsheets	☐	☐	☐
Sending an email	☐	☐	☐
Using the Internet	☐	☐	☐

The SEQ is © UMD Professional Ltd.

Appendix 4
The structure of the appraisal meeting

Stage	Person being appraised	Appraiser	Comments
1 Overview	How would you describe your achievements in the past year?	How would the appraiser describe the dentist's achievements in the past year?	The areas that 'achievements' refers to will have been previously agreed. They may relate to the dentist as individual/clinician/team member.
2 Positive evaluation	With regard to these areas, what did you do well? How do you know?	What did the dentist do well? How does the appraiser know? (Which of the previously agreed objectives in the PDP were met? What is the feedback from the team?)	The appraisee should state the evaluation tools that he used, e.g. data collection, audit, self-evaluations, questionnaires, etc. The appraiser should discuss any positive feedback that has been received, using specific examples whenever possible.

Stage	Person being appraised	Appraiser	Comments
3 Personal development needs	What did not go well? Deriving from these areas, what personal development needs do you have? How do you know?	What did not go well? How does the appraiser know? (Were previously agreed objectives met? What is the feedback from the team if this has been sought?)	To avoid this stage becoming negative and to maintain trust, ensure that honest but constructive comments are made. The appraiser should discuss any negative feedback that has been received using specific examples and any suggestions made by contributors. The appraiser should not dictate, but encourage the appraisee to suggest improvements. Personal development needs may be derived from performance as an individual/clinician/team member and may reflect personal ambitions, CPD needs and service needs.
4 Objectives for change	Which areas for improvement do you wish to prioritise?	Appraiser's comments.	The appraiser and appraisee should jointly decide upon two or three specific objectives to be achieved before the next appraisal meeting. They must be feasible.
5 Practical planning	What resources will you require?	Appraiser's comments.	In broad terms, the resources should be identified so that a start can be made. A proforma might be completed at this stage (*see* Appendix 5).

Appendix 5
Summary of the appraisal meeting

Dentist:	Appraiser:	Date:

Stage	*Summary*
Overview	
Positive evaluation	
Personal development needs	
Objectives for change	
Practical planning (e.g. resources)	

Date of next appraisal:

Appendix 6
GDP 360° feedback form

Dentist: Date:

Do not write your name, but which team are you a member of?
(This question can be omitted where the team is small.)

Questions 1–23 and the very end of this document should be answered by everyone. Please encircle *one* number for those questions that you feel you *can* answer.

  Remember to be honest, but not deliberately hurtful. Give positive feedback if this is appropriate, but where it is not, please suggest *how* the dentist might improve.

Area			
Communication	*Score /80*	*Scale*	*Comments/specific examples*
The dentist:		1 = totally disagree	
		10 = totally agree	
1 Is approachable		1 2 3 4 5 6 7 8 9 10	
2 Speaks courteously to the staff		1 2 3 4 5 6 7 8 9 10	
3 Communicates clearly verbally and in writing		1 2 3 4 5 6 7 8 9 10	
4 Shows willingness to explain where necessary		1 2 3 4 5 6 7 8 9 10	
5 Listens to the staff		1 2 3 4 5 6 7 8 9 10	
6 Asks about the staff members' point of view		1 2 3 4 5 6 7 8 9 10	
7 Keeps the staff informed about issues relevant to them		1 2 3 4 5 6 7 8 9 10	
8 Responds promptly to messages		1 2 3 4 5 6 7 8 9 10	

Motivation   Score   /50

The dentist:

9 Shows enthusiasm for his work   1 2 3 4 5 6 7 8 9 10

10 Appears willing to take on new ideas   1 2 3 4 5 6 7 8 9 10

11 Encourages others to have a positive approach to their   1 2 3 4 5 6 7 8 9 10
   work

12 Recognises the achievements of others   1 2 3 4 5 6 7 8 9 10

13 Supports the professional development of others   1 2 3 4 5 6 7 8 9 10

Time management/stress   Score   /40

The dentist:

14 Is punctual in arrival   1 2 3 4 5 6 7 8 9 10

15 Keeps to appointment times in surgeries   1 2 3 4 5 6 7 8 9 10

16 Appears to cope well with stress   1 2 3 4 5 6 7 8 9 10

17 Recognises and responds when staff members are   1 2 3 4 5 6 7 8 9 10
   under stress

As a working colleague Score /60

The dentist:

18 Delegates to the appropriate person   1 2 3 4 5 6 7 8 9 10

19 Only expects immediate action from staff where this is appropriate   1 2 3 4 5 6 7 8 9 10

20 Chooses an appropriate time and place to address issues   1 2 3 4 5 6 7 8 9 10

21 Obeys agreed protocols   1 2 3 4 5 6 7 8 9 10

22 Makes himself available to answer the staff's queries   1 2 3 4 5 6 7 8 9 10

23 Responds courteously to requests for assistance   1 2 3 4 5 6 7 8 9 10

The following questions should also be answered by the dentists.

Care of patients Score /60

24 Treats patients politely and with consideration   1 2 3 4 5 6 7 8 9 10

25 Makes efforts to ensure that the patient has understood his condition, its treatment and prognosis   1 2 3 4 5 6 7 8 9 10

26 Takes care to preserve the patient's privacy and dignity   1 2 3 4 5 6 7 8 9 10

27 Obtains informed consent to treatment   1 2 3 4 5 6 7 8 9 10

28 Involves patients in decisions about their care   1 2 3 4 5 6 7 8 9 10

29 Keeps patients' information confidential   1 2 3 4 5 6 7 8 9 10

Ethical standards   Score /30

30 Does not impose his own beliefs and values   1 2 3 4 5 6 7 8 9 10

31 Does not show prejudice   1 2 3 4 5 6 7 8 9 10

32 Does not seek or accept financial rewards from patients outside the normal framework of professional fees   1 2 3 4 5 6 7 8 9 10

Clinical standards   Score /60

33 Makes appropriate management plans   1 2 3 4 5 6 7 8 9 10

34 Makes appropriate referrals   1 2 3 4 5 6 7 8 9 10

35 Prescribes appropriately   1 2 3 4 5 6 7 8 9 10

36 Accepts responsibility for own actions and decisions   1 2 3 4 5 6 7 8 9 10

37 Records each patient contact   1 2 3 4 5 6 7 8 9 10

38 Keeps sufficient records to allow another practitioner to continue the patient's care   1 2 3 4 5 6 7 8 9 10

Maintaining standards   Score /30

39 Monitors his own performance   1 2 3 4 5 6 7 8 9 10

40 Reports near misses and significant events   1 2 3 4 5 6 7 8 9 10

41 Undertakes continuing professional development   1 2 3 4 5 6 7 8 9 10

As a partner   Score /30

The dentist:

42 Adequately discharges his partnership responsibilities   1 2 3 4 5 6 7 8 9 10

43 Is willing to accept new responsibilities   1 2 3 4 5 6 7 8 9 10

44 Provides positive support to colleagues who have made mistakes or whose performance gives cause for concern   1 2 3 4 5 6 7 8 9 10

Wider professional duties   Score /20

The dentist:

45 Adequately discharges his teaching/educational responsibilities   1 2 3 4 5 6 7 8 9 10

46 Contributes to the wider development of the profession   1 2 3 4 5 6 7 8 9 10

If you wish, please add any comments on areas not referred to above.

What do you most value about this colleague?

Thank you for your time. Please leave the completed form in the envelope in the dentist's message box.

Index